The Nurse's Communication Advantage

How Business-Savvy Communication Skills Can Advance your Nursing Career

By Kathleen D. Pagana, PhD, RN

Sigma Theta Tau International
Honor Society of Nursing®

Sigma Theta Tau International

Sigma Theta Tau International
550 West North Street
Indianapolis, IN 46202

To order additional books, buy in bulk, or order for corporate use, contact Nursing Knowledge International at 888.NKI.4YOU (888.654.4968/US and Canada) or +1.317.634.8171 (outside US and Canada).

To request a review copy for course adoption, e-mail solutions@nursingknowledge.org or call 888.NKI.4YOU (888.654.4968/US and Canada) or +1.317.917.4983 (outside US and Canada).

To request author information, or for speaker or other media requests, contact Rachael McLaughlin of the Honor Society of Nursing, Sigma Theta Tau International at 888.634.7575 (US and Canada) or +1.317.634.8171 (outside US and Canada).

ISBN-13: 978-1-930538-96-2

Library of Congress Cataloging-in-Publication Data

Pagana, Kathleen Deska, 1952-
  The nurse's communication advantage / Kathleen Pagana.
       p. ; cm.
  Includes bibliographical references and index.
  ISBN 978-1-930538-96-2 (alk. paper)
  1. Communication in nursing. I. Sigma Theta Tau International. II.
Title.
  [DNLM: 1. Nursing. 2. Communication. 3. Nurse-Patient Relations. 4.
Vocational Guidance. WY 16.1]
  RT23.P335 2010
  610.7306'99--dc22
                                                                2010027642

First Printing, 2010

Publisher: Renee Wilmeth
Acquisitions Editor: Cynthia Saver, RN, MS, and Janet Boivin, RN
Editorial Coordinator: Paula Jeffers
Cover Designer: Studio Galou
Interior Design and Page Composition: Rebecca Batchelor

Principal Editor: Carla Hall
Copy Editor: Brian Walls
Proofreader: Barbara Bennett
Indexer: Jane Palmer
Illustrator: Amanda Emig

Dedication

This book is dedicated with love and appreciation to my mother, Margaret Kathleen McDermott Deska, who fostered my love of learning from a very young age. Her children and grandchildren will never forget her support for education and learning which is depicted in her favorite expression:

"Take care of your books and your books will take care of you."

Acknowledgements

This book would not have been possible without the support and encouragement from many people from many different points in my life. I will always be thankful and appreciative for my parents (Edward and Margaret Deska) who gave me "roots to grow and wings to fly." Without a doubt, I am forever indebted to the many good teachers and professors who inspired me and gave me the confidence to pursue my dreams.

As with everything in my life, my husband (Timothy J. Pagana) has been my best and most enthusiastic source of support. I would also like to thank Marjorie Brody from Brody Professionals for her guidance and the opportunity she gave me at an important transitional point in my life. Finally, I would like to acknowledge and thank Cindy Saver, Renee Wilmeth, Janet Boivin, Carla Hall, and everyone else at Sigma Theta Tau International for their enthusiastic support of this book.

About the Author

Kathleen D. Pagana, PhD, RN, is a dynamic speaker and an accomplished author. She is a professor emeritus at Lycoming College in Williamsport, Pennsylvania, and the president of Pagana Keynotes & Presentations. She has been a leader in health care for more than 30 years. She has a BSN from the University of Maryland and a MSN and PhD in nursing from the University of Pennsylvania.

Pagana is the author of more than 75 articles and 25 books. More than one million copies of *Mosby's Diagnostic and Laboratory Test Reference,* and *Mosby's Manual of Diagnostic and Laboratory Tests,* have sold worldwide, with translations in French, Chinese, Korean, Spanish, and Portuguese. She is the author of *The Nurse's Etiquette Advantage: How Professional Etiquette Can Advance Your Nursing Career.* She is on the editorial boards of *AORN Journal* and *Nurse Educator.* Her most prestigious awards include the Army Commendation Medal, a Faculty Award for Teaching Excellence, and numerous accolades recognizing her articles and books.

From her experiences as a patient care manager, military officer, faculty chair, academic dean, professional speaker, and consultant, she has recognized and learned the vital necessity for strong business communication skills. Being a member of the board of directors of a regional medical center has helped Kathy understand the complexity of health care and the ongoing challenges for nurse leaders and managers. She keeps current in clinical practice and connected with nurses at the bedside by working several days a month in a hospital.

She has enjoyed the privilege of helping thousands of people around the world improve their communication skills and feel more confident in both business and social situations. Pagana speaks nationally and internationally on the challenges of leadership, communication, professional etiquette, and life balance. She can be contacted on her website at www.KathleenPagana.com or by e-mailing her at Kathy@KathleenPagana.com.

Table of Contents

Foreword

If you knew that you could motivate others to make a difference, would you be willing to try? If you discovered that you possess leadership qualities and skills, would you share them?

Kathleen Pagana does both with this important new book, *The Nurse's Communication Advantage*. At every stage of their careers, nurses will find the content of this book vital for establishing, building, and improving their professional relationships. This excellent handbook offers nurses unique, practical, and straight-forward advice on business communication skills.

As a nurse executive in the business world, I am often asked by nurses just starting out in their careers how I got to my current station of leadership, and what education it took to get me into the boardrooms of some of the top health establishments in the world. I answer them with a very short list of requirements: hard work, persistence, and excellent communication skills! As I climbed the clinical ladder at the National Institutes of Health and then transitioned into television and global health initiatives, I had to navigate the turbulent waters of the corporate media realm with no preparedness in business communication. My path would have been made infinitely easier with *The Nurse's Communication Advantage* in my library.

Kathleen Pagana outlines a comprehensive set of communication guidelines on a wide range of situations, from presentation skills and written communication to development of useful networks and cross-generational communications. Whether the issue is cultural communication barriers, social media, or e-mail etiquette, Kathleen Pagana delivers the keys to success.

The Nurse's Communication Advantage delivers the communication skills all nurses need for success. With this excellent foundation, each nurse will be motivated to join the trailblazers who have gone before.

I challenge you to continue your important work with the words of Ralph Waldo Emerson: "Do not go where the path may lead; go instead where there is no path and leave a trail."

—Donna Hill Howes, RN, MS
Senior Vice President, Sharecare

Introduction

At a recent nursing conference, a speaker lamented, "Nursing 101 did not provide the business savvy needed for successful navigation of a nursing career." How true that is — especially for business communication! Although nurses learn a lot about patient communication, many (or most) have a knowledge deficit when it comes to business communication. Just doing your job doesn't mean you'll move ahead in your career. You need to stand out.

Effective business communication can provide the edge you need for career development and advancement. This idea is supported by subscribers of the *Harvard Business Review* who noted, "The ability to communicate was rated as the most important factor in making a manager 'promotable'" (Blalock, 2005). According to Steve Adubato, the most successful professionals are those with the best relationships. He noted that although these people may not have the best intellects, they always are the best communicators (2007).

Why is business communication important for nursing? Flatter organizations, employee diversity, and greater use of teams have made business communication essential to the success of organizations. The autocratic management of the past is being replaced by participatory management in which communication is needed to build trust, promote understanding, and empower others (Blalock, 2005). A good example of this is the shared governance component of Magnet Hospitals.

Business communication skills can make or break a career. Many talented and ambitious nurses fail to achieve their potential because they have not mastered the art of effective business communication. In a fun and easy-to-read manner, this book targets the needs and interests of nurses in various phases of career growth. For example, this book can help you in the following situations:

* Developing strong networks
* Improving interdisciplinary communication
* Developing powerful presentation skills

* Writing business memos and reports

* Using e-mail in a professional and courteous manner

* Writing an article for publication

* Facilitating productive meetings

* Communicating across generations

* Utilizing social media

* Overcoming cultural communication barriers

Key Features

Many engaging text features encourage active reader participation and make this book an indispensible guide for nurses. The writing style is fun and informative. The following are some of the other key features of *The Nurse's Communication Advantage*.

①

A unique feature of this book is its organization in a "question and answer" format.

This is an example of how the question of the Q&A format will look.

This is what the answer of the Q&A format will look like.

③

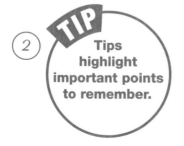

② **Tips highlight important points to remember.**

Communication Coach

Communication Coach sidebar boxes provide anecdotes showing positive and negative business communication scenarios with a take-home lesson.

Tables help itemize and illustrate information.

(4) This is what a table will look like in the book

Column 1 Heading	Column 2 Heading
Column 1 data will be here	Column 2 data will be here

(5)

Inspirational quotes are sprinkled throughout the book. They will motivate and inspire you!

✔ *Checklist* **(6)**

Chapter Checklists are provided at the end of each chapter. These checklists provide a means for the reader to review key points and assess learning.

(7)

? Frequently Asked Questions (FAQ) and answers are included in each chapter.

(8) TAKE-AWAY TIPS

Each chapter ends with Take-Away Tips. These are the types of tips you'll want hanging on your bulletin board to read and re-read every day.

New professionals will find this book a vital component for building their careers, and experienced professionals will enjoy this not-to-be missed review and update. For some nurses, presentation skills will be a critical link to career advancement. For others, writing skills will be a priority; incorporating social media may provide an edge for surviving, but also thriving. *The Nurse's Communication Advantage* is filled with practical insights that can boost the credibility of nurses

Whether it's getting a mentor or getting on Facebook, the skills presented in this book can nourish any career. Effective business communication skills are not optional for career development and advancement. You can benefit every day — in business and personal encounters — by using *The Nurse's Communication Advantage* to present yourself as confident, polished, and professional.

P.S. Before you get started, don't forget to take the business communication quiz on page xvii to test your knowledge. The answers are in the back of the book.

Quiz: Business Communication

Test Your Knowledge Questions

1. Participation in sports provides an edge in the business world.

   True   False

2. There are differences in the way men and women often handle complaints.

   True   False

3. Start every speech thanking the audience for inviting you to speak.

   True   False

4. Any story is an asset to a presentation.

   True   False

5. There is an easy way to "blank or blacken" the screen during a PowerPoint presentation.

   True   False

6. Use the blind carbon copy (Bcc) when sending an e-mail to a list of unrelated people.

   True   False

7. Emoticons are acceptable to use in a business e-mail.

   True   False

8. Always send a query letter to a journal editor.

   True   False

9. Anyone who helps you write an article should be listed as a co-author.

   True   False

10. Before calling a meeting, determine if the meeting is really necessary.

    True   False

11. Workers from Generation Y (Gen Yers) require a lot of feedback on the job.

    True   False

12. Employers can use LinkedIn to get background information on job candidates.

    True   False

13. Blogs are more engaging than websites.

    True   False

14. Search engines rank websites higher than blogs.

    True   False

15. Twitter asks the question, "What are you doing?"

    True   False

16. Be careful of what you post on Facebook.

    True   False

17. Being "a little late" has different connotations around the world.

    True   False

18. The meaning of the "okay" sign is the same around the world.

    True   False

19. Smiling is a universal gesture of happiness.

    True   False

20. In an international setting, gifts are always appreciated.

    True   False

1

✳

Building Relationships

Do you:

Know how to build a strong network?

Wonder how to make your team more effective?

Need to improve your listening skills?

Know how to improve communications with people from other disciplines?

Understand gender differences in communication styles?

Put your best foot forward in your professional setting?

When you get right down to it, business is all about relationships. Who you know and the relationships you develop impact your success. Often, the soft skills make the hard difference in business decisions.

Knowing the importance of networks, teams, listening skills, interdisciplinary communication, and gender variations in communication can help you put your best foot forward in any business setting.

"The vacuum created by a failure to communicate will quickly be filled with rumor, misrepresentations, drivel, and poison."

–C. Northcote Parkinson

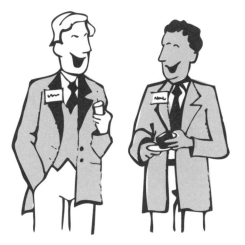

Developing a Strong Network

How important is a strong network?

There is no denying that networking works. With a strong network, a person has many more opportunities and relationships. Business gets done through relationships. It isn't enough to do a job well. Accept networking as an integral part of your job that benefits you and your company.

"People buy people' before they buy services and products."

–Will Kintish

What are some ideas for expanding your network?

Here are some suggestions:

* Focus on being a resource for others rather than on your own agenda.

* Join organizations and associations.

* Attend professional meetings and conferences.

* Serve on committees.

* Volunteer in your community.

* Participate in local sports by joining a golf team, a running group, or a softball league.

* Attend cocktail receptions.

* Join a health club or gym.

* Make use of social media, such as LinkedIn and Facebook (See Chapter 8).

How can you nurture your relationships?

Networking requires an ongoing process of outreach and maintenance to build and nurture relationships. Look for ways to connect with people. Send notes, meet for lunch, and acknowledge accomplishments. Send information (articles, websites, etc.) to someone who could use it. Don't just connect when you need a favor. Thank people for helping you.

TIP

Make the first move when meeting new people.

How can networking help your career?

Although many people use networking to enhance their career opportunities, it has many other rewards (Shepard & Stimmler, 2005):

* Learning interpersonal and leadership skills

* Acquiring valuable information

* Becoming known and liked

* Developing business relationships

* Solving problems and brainstorming ideas

* Being invited to join a board or committee

* Learning about new business opportunities

* Broadening your sphere of influence

* Helping others

* Having fun and making friends

Communication Coach

Rosemary and Bonnie were chatting before their yoga class. Because their children had been in school together since kindergarten, Bonnie was sharing her disappointment regarding her son not getting a job after interviewing at a pharmaceutical company. When Rosemary heard the name of the company, she said she was very familiar with the company because she teaches business etiquette there as part of the sales academy for new employees. After Rosemary contacted the director, Bonnie's son received a call for another interview and got the job.

Lesson: Networking can occur in any setting. Don't underestimate its power.

Team Building

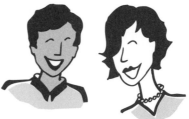

"Teamwork gives you the best opportunity to turn your vision into reality."

–John C. Maxwell

Why is team building so important?

Achieving success requires more than technical skills and knowledge. It requires people skills and the ability to work in teams.

Most of what goes on in a work setting takes place in teams. Often, one reason smart and talented people don't succeed in the workplace is because they are either unwilling or unable to work in teams. Team players need to be good communicators. They especially need to listen to each other in order to succeed. Good talkers can be the worst team players.

What are some characteristics of effective teams?

Effective teams require members to do the following (Adubato, 2006):

* Know the team's goal.

* Understand how their role relates to the overall success of the team.

* Have the necessary tools to fulfill their roles.

* Support a collegial environment that encourages candid dialogue.

* Be willing to take risks and suggest ideas without the fear of reprisal.

* Trust each other.

* Have an "all-for-one-and-one-for-all" mentality.

* Encourage feedback.

* Treat each other in a civil and respectful manner.

Heinemann and Zeiss (2002) describe the "12 C's of teamwork." Interactions guided by these principles can produce creative synergies among members and result in new and unexpected ideas and solutions. These 12 principles include

1. Communication

2. Cooperation

3. Cohesiveness

4. Commitment

5. Collaboration

6. Confronts problems directly

7. Coordination of effort

8. Conflict management

9. Consensus decision making

10. Caring

11. Consistency (with one another)

12. Contribution

Communication Coach

In the movie *Rocky,* boxer Rocky Balboa describes his relationship with his girlfriend, Adrien. "I've got gaps. She's got gaps. But together we've got no gaps."

Lesson: This is a great description of teamwork. Teamwork can help us handle our weaknesses (Maxwell, 2007).

Why is teamwork essential for health care delivery?

Biomedical advances, the aging population, and regulatory and cost containment measures have increased the complexity of health care. As a result, the boundaries between health care professionals have blurred, and the need for interdependence has increased. Additionally, better teamwork can increase job satisfaction and retention and lower burnout (Rafferty, Ball, & Aiken, 2001).

How can conflict, if managed correctly, be desirable in a group?

Without conflict, groupthink can result where creative, contradictory ideas are suppressed in the interest of maintaining consensus and peaceful relationships. Healthy conflict is a sign that diverse ideas are welcome (Lindeke & Sieckert, 2005).

How about team leadership?

Every team should have a primary leader who sets the tone and fosters the environment of individual growth and team success. However, any team member should be able to step up and become a situational leader at any time. This flexibility in the team structure is critical for success (Adubato, 2006).

Does participation in sports give men an advantage in being team players?

Yes. Before women got involved in sports, men learned (as boys) the importance of teamwork. Today, men and women both have this learning opportunity. Many valuable lessons from participation in team sports can apply in business. Some examples include the following:

* ✳ The importance of competition

* ✳ How to win and lose

* ✳ That cooperation is necessary

* ✳ If you get knocked down, you have to get back up

* ✳ How to take criticism

* ✳ The good feeling from being part of something bigger than yourself (Tracy, 2001).

Learning to Listen and Listening to Learn

"Listening, not imitation, may be the sincerest form of flattery."

–Dr. Joyce Brothers

Why is it important to have good listening skills?

Listening is a key element for developing and sustaining relationships. How we listen and respond to others influences how others respond to us. When people feel listened to, they're more likely to share ideas and thoughts. Table 1.1 provides some good tips on listening:

1.1 Tips for Good Listening

Things to Do	Things to Avoid
Make good eye contact	Finishing sentences
Ignore distractions	Daydreaming
Smile and nod your head	Interrupting
Ask relevant questions	Changing the subject
Face the person	Distracting body language
Lean forward	Looking at your watch, PDA, or iPhone
Keep an open mind	Making assumptions or prejudgments
Be present and focused	Filling "airtime"

(Pagana, 2008)

Can you give some examples of how people communicate in ways that inhibit positive relationships?

Yes. Here are six common listening misbehaviors (Eichhorn, Thomas-Maddox, & Wanzer, 2008):

1. Pseudo-listening: Listeners pretend to be listening when they are not.

2. Monopolizing: Listeners take the focus off the speaker and redirect the conversation to them.

3. Disconfirming: Listeners deny the feelings of others by saying things like, "There's no need to cry."

4. Defensive listening: In this situation, listeners perceive a threatening environment. For example, "I didn't tell you to do that."

5. Selective listening: Listeners focus on only parts of the message and respond only to those.

6. Ambushing: Listeners use information they hear to attack the speaker.

What should you do if you miss an important part of a conversation?

Say, "I'm sorry. I missed that. Would you please repeat what you just said?" This is better than faking your way through a concentration lapse and playing catch-up after you return to the conversation.

"It's a tossup as to which are finally the most exasperating—the dull people who never talk or the bright people who never listen."

–Sydney Harris

Communication Coach

Rusty and Jane were cleaning up the kitchen after eating dinner. Jane was upset and described some comments written by her supervisor on her annual review. Rusty gave a halfhearted response while peering at the TV in the family room. Jane scolded Rusty for not listening to her. Rusty was shocked and said, "What do you mean? I heard every word you said." Jane countered with, "Prove it! What did I just say?" Rusty dropped his head and apologized, realizing that while he had heard Jane talking, he hadn't really listened to a word she said.

Lesson: A common mistake in the listening process is to assume that hearing is the same as listening.

How do you handle a conversation when someone says something unusual or unflattering?

Listen for motives. People often reveal what they really think by denying it. For example, suppose a manager says, "I'm not a dictator, but I do have high standards." Likely, some people have told him that he is a dictator and he is bothered by this. You could foster your relationship by helping him picture himself as a strict but fair leader (Soden, 1996).

"People do business with people they know, like, and trust."

–Susan RoAnn

Interdisciplinary Communication

"The meaning of your communication is the response you get."

–John Bandler and Richard Grinder

Why is interdisciplinary communication an essential component of health care communication?

Each health care professional has information that others need to practice successfully. As a result, effective communication needs to cross several relevant disciplines to achieve favorable patient outcomes. Research with Magnet hospitals has shown that healthy collaboration between nurses and doctors is directly linked to optimal patient outcomes (Kirchheimer, 2010; Kramer & Schmalenberg, 2008).

If they have questions or concerns about patient care, health care professionals need to feel they can speak openly without fear of reprisal or embarrassment. Mistakes in health care are often blamed on the failure of interdisciplinary communication. This communication is essential not only for the benefit of patients, but also for the satisfaction of health care providers (Lindeke & Sieckert, 2005; Rafferty, Ball, & Aiken, 2001; Reeder, 2007).

Communication Coach

Cheri worked with a doctor that her colleagues described as a "terror." One afternoon, she overhead the doctor making disparaging remarks about nursing care to one of her patients. She made an appointment with him in his office for the next morning. She explained her role as a primary nurse and emphasized the importance of partnering with him and other health care providers. After that meeting, this doctor started to ask for Cheri's opinion about patient care issues and requested to have his patients admitted to her block.

Lesson: If you act like a professional, you will be treated with respect. When you are frustrated, take responsibility for finding a solution.

What are some factors that can produce different perspectives on communication?

There are a number of factors that can impact communication between nurses and physicians. Some examples include the following (Reader, 2007):

* Hierarchical factors

* Gender

* Different patient care responsibilities

* Differences in training methods of nurses and doctors.

* Disputes over boundaries of authority

How can understanding and tolerance of different interdisciplinary perspectives support patient care?

Collaboration among individuals with different skill sets can result in creative and practical solutions that otherwise would not occur. For this reason, professionals should avoid making assumptions about other professionals and take the time and effort to learn from each other.

How can technology improve interdisciplinary communication?

Electronic and wireless forms of communication can promote more frequent and easier contact with colleagues, improve access to data necessary for patient care, and improve documentation of interdisciplinary communication. These factors all improve working relationships (Dykes, 2006).

Gender Differences in Communication

Are there gender differences in communication?

Yes, but.... It's wise to be aware of some common differences, but remember there are probably as many differences within the sexes as between them. Be careful of making widespread generalizations. Gender stereotypes are becoming dead and obsolete. More and more women communicate in an assertive manner, and many men communicate in a compassionate and caring manner (Adubato, 2006).

Keep in mind that differences in communication are a matter of degree. Also, differences do not exist in all men and women. No one communication style is better than the other, just different.

What are some of the differences in the communication styles of men and women?

One difference may relate to the way the two sexes display their expertise. Because women seek to build rapport, they often downplay their expertise rather than display it. However, because men value the feeling of knowing more and taking center stage, they seek opportunities to display their expertise (Tannen, 1990).

When stressed, men will often stand up, look eye to eye, and attempt to intimidate physically. Due to a size disparity, women do not do that. What women can do is discuss what the man is doing and encourage a less hostile mood to facilitate resolution.

What is the potential impact of taking things personally?

Many women do this and live in a state of anxiety and turmoil because of it. They may need to toughen up a bit. This is hard for women, because they often build their lives around relationships. In contrast, men build their lives around achievement. Instead of taking the annoying behaviors of others as personal affronts, women need to look at these behaviors as part of the gamesmanship that goes on in companies (Tracy, 2001). They need to be more objective when dealing with the issue and aim for a resolution.

What can you learn about the opposite sex by listening to their conversation?

You can learn a lot. For example, suppose you are talking with Mike about a building proposal and Joe joins in and starts talking about football. Listen carefully. Do they admire team players or focus on individual players? Do they praise risky offensive plays? The qualities they admire in sports are probably the same as those they admire in business.

Let's take another example. Suppose you overhear Denise and Theresa talking about Denise's upcoming wedding. Is Denise organized or haphazard in her planning? Is she concerned about insulting people who are not invited? Is she stressed out? These are all clues to her personality, values, and organizational skills.

Do men and women handle complaints differently?

Yes. When women complain to a peer, they often want empathy, not advice. In contrast, men don't want to empathize as much as they want to fix the problem (Shipley & Schwalbe, 2007). You can see how these different approaches may not be appreciated or valued by the opposite sex.

How do women and men differ in the way they report information?

Women like to discuss people, setting, context, and inner meaning. Men usually skim the surface. The detailed reporting style of women is often viewed by men as "rambling." If women don't understand this difference and make adjustments, they may not understand why some corporate doors are closed to them (Shepard & Stimmler, 2005).

Generally, stick to the facts that are important and relevant to the issue. Offer the details as an option. If no one wants the details, you've saved yourself and others time.

Are there other traits of women that can have a negative connotation in the business world?

Yes. Shepard and Stimmler (2005) have identified a number of characteristics that are in this "catch-22" category. See Table 1.2 for some examples.

1.2 — The "Catch-22" Corporate Communication Chart

Traits of Women	Possible Interpretation by Men
Women are good listeners.	Women are passive and don't have strong opinions.
Women are serious about their work.	Women lack a sense of humor.
Women like to solicit feedback from others.	Women are indecisive.
Women use body language to encourage speakers.	Women's behavior can be interpreted as agreement.
Women raise their voices to be heard.	Women are too aggressive.
Women politely wait to be called upon in a meeting.	Women are weak.

Aren't there communication traits of women that would be beneficial for men to learn or improve?

Yes, there sure are. If you look at the "Catch-22" Corporate Communication Chart, men would only stand to benefit by practicing some of the traits listed, such as listening better, soliciting feedback, and being more polite. Please remember that gender-related communication stereotypes are becoming obsolete.

Why are some women criticized for frequently apologizing and saying "I'm sorry?"

They are criticized because it looks like they are putting themselves down. However, often the apology does not mean accepting blame as much as it shows concern about someone's feelings. For example, saying "I'm sorry" when someone breaks a leg means, "I'm sorry it happened."

Negative impressions result from situations when some people use frequent apologies and others do not. Frequent apologizers may be disagreeing with a statement or may seem to be taking blame for mishaps that are not their fault. Women are more likely to do this than men (Tannen, 1994).

What are some alternatives to replace the habit of apologizing?

Instead of saying "I'm sorry," "Excuse me, but," or "I may be wrong, but," simply state your opinion. If you need an introduction, say, "With all due respect..." Like any other habit, the habit of apologizing can be broken with awareness and practice.

Communication Coach

Monica was meeting with five men in a brainstorming session. During the hour-long meeting, Monica repeatedly said, "I'm sorry" or "I apologize." Everyone made corrections and additions. None of the men ever apologized. None of them had any more reason to apologize than she did.

Lesson: The reason Monica's frequent apologies stood out was that she was the only person apologizing. These ritual apologies may impact her perceived level of confidence or competence.

Do men and women have different styles of humor?

Men generally find poking-fun at others funny, while women prefer situational humor, such as self-deprecating anecdotes (RoAnn, 2000). Men often think teasing is funny, whereas women are more likely to take it personally (Shipley & Schwalbe, 2007).

Men tease people they like as well as people they don't like. They often "clown around" to break tension and decrease embarrassment.

How should women respond to humor in the workplace?

Women should show their sense of humor by participating in or showing appreciation for appropriate banter and jokes. When women are included in jokes, it often means they are part of the team. Smiling or laughing can generate good will and establish rapport (Shepard & Stimmler, 2005).

This does not apply to racist or off-color jokes. An appropriate response may be, "Let's not go there."

> *"Many a true word is spoken in jest."*
>
> –Proverbial truth, first attributed to Chaucer

Can you recommend some tips for enhancing communication between the sexes?

Yes. Treat men and women as professionals and talented employees rather than as stereotypical men and women. Try to understand and celebrate gender differences. Here are some tips to improve communication (Lindsell-Roberts, 2000):

* A female isn't a dame, a chick, or a girl. It is better to say, "There are two women working in marketing" rather than, "There are two girls."

* Use gender-neutral terms as much as possible when appropriate. For instance, *staffing* the booth is just as understandable as *manning* the booth.

* That said, women should avoid getting hung up on every word that may appear sexist. Complaining about words like *sportsmanship* or *manpower* doesn't accomplish much.

* Avoid creating an uncomfortable environment by telling off-color jokes, using offensive language, commenting on a person's physical attributes, using demeaning nicknames, or discussing sexual activities.

* Don't repeat or engage in gossip.

* Be tactful when offering criticism. Do it privately.

* Accept compliments graciously and say, "Thank you."

* If you want to be treated as a professional, make sure you dress like one.

* Show respect, courtesy, and consideration for the feelings of others.

Communication Coach

Brian and his wife, Ellen, were pulling into a parking lot at a local restaurant. When Brian saw one of his friends walking across the parking lot, he sped up the car and almost ran into his friend. Brian thought this was really funny. His wife did not. She thought it was mean-spirited and could have caused injury.

Lesson: Men and women have different ideas of humor.

Putting Your Best Foot Forward

"If I am not for myself, who will be?"

—The Talmud

How can you demonstrate your expertise in an effective way?

Here are some suggestions to put your best self forward (Shepard & Stimmler, 2005):

* Keep a list of the skills you use to achieve success in the forefront of your mind. Refer to it when the

opportunity presents itself. (For example, "I like and enjoy the challenge of writing and articulating ideas.")

* Link your skills to your experience and be able to describe your accomplishments in a sentence or two. (For example, "Writing articles on business etiquette was vitally important for securing my book contract.")

* Demonstrate your leadership qualities and don't be afraid to use the "I" word. Promoting yourself and praising your team leads to better recognition for all. (For example, "I and my competent team members are drafting the proposal on shared governance.")

* Promote yourself with subtlety and finesse. (For example, "My new book received a great review in the *AORN Journal*.") Don't brag about yourself.

How can you demonstrate your interest in lifelong learning?

Be teachable. Be engaged and excited about learning. Make sure your attitude demonstrates your interest in discovery, discussion, growth, and applying new information. There is a relationship between passion and potential (Maxwell, 2007).

What is the best way to handle feedback?

Invite candid feedback about your performance. Be humble and embrace feedback. Don't let pride close your mind to welcoming feedback. Understanding, analyzing, and acting on feedback requires wisdom.

What are some tips for setting and meeting goals?

Believe in your goals and visualize what is required to achieve them. Be willing to pay the price. Goals are invaluable for success, especially if they are SMART goals as described in the following list (Acuff & Wood, 2004):

* **S**pecific—Avoid vague and nebulous goals. For example, "I want to live in a condo near the Art Museum in Philadelphia" is specific.

* **M**easureable—Shows you are reaching your goal or making progress.

* **A**chievable—Challenging, but attainable.

* **R**ealistic—You have the skills and resources to reach the goal within a specified time period.

* **T**ime-sensitive—There is an endpoint or deadline for meeting the goal.

"The future belongs to those who believe in the beauty of their dreams."

–Eleanor Roosevelt

What's the benefit of having a mentor?

Mentors can provide the wisdom, knowledge, and understanding that might otherwise take years to learn on your own. As such, mentors accelerate your learning curve and steer you in the right direction. Mentors can help support your ideas, introduce you to the right people, and help you build a network of support and influence. In essence, they can help you discover and make full use of your personal potential.

How do you find a mentor?

Sometimes mentoring relationships occur naturally. For example, you might connect with someone you met in the interview or orientation process. In some cases, you may be assigned a mentor through a mentoring program. Other times, you have to actively look for a mentor. Here are some questions to guide your selection of a mentor (Klaus, 2007):

* Do I like and respect the person?
* Does the person have stature within the organization?
* Is the person experienced with the company?
* Has the person advocated for you or others?
* Is the person held in high regard by others?
* Do you think you can trust the person?

Why would a busy, successful person agree to be a mentor?

Many people are flattered when someone asks them to be a mentor. Often, these mentors were mentored by someone else and are successful because of that. They enjoy the privilege of giving back and fostering the development of others.

Do you have any suggestions for initiating contact with a potential mentor?

It is a good idea to test the potential relationship by getting together in an informal setting, such as going out for coffee or lunch. If you feel comfortable with the person, explain your reason for getting together and how much you would appreciate advice on an ongoing basis. If the person is interested, discuss potential time commitments and expectations for the relationship (Klaus, 2007).

"A human being is like a delicate instrument that must be kept under the right conditions and constantly fine-tuned."

–Diane Tracy

How important is business etiquette for career success?

Business etiquette is not optional for personal and professional success—it's a necessity.

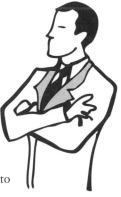

Anyone can become an expert in etiquette. Etiquette is like a sport. If you have the skills to play, people will want you on their team. The more skilled you are, the more you will be offered opportunities and positions. Here are some key etiquette tips related to business communication (Pagana, 2008):

* Create a positive and confident impression with your handshake.

* Introduce yourself to those you don't know.

* Learn to remember names.

* Wear your name badge on the right-hand side of your chest so it is more easily seen when shaking hands.

* Be courteous to everyone.

* Always listen intently to others.

* Speak so you can be easily heard, but not too loudly.

* Be aware of the impact of body language on communication.

* Find out what people want and help them get it.

* Seek to understand the other person's point of view.

* Thank people for their input and help.

* Acknowledge a compliment with a smile and a "Thank you."

* Write thank-you notes.

* If you forgot to send a thank-you note, send it late. Late is better than never.

✳ Use proper grammar and spelling.

✳ Meet deadlines and respond to RSVPs.

✔ *Checklist*

Building Relationships

❑ Do I have an example demonstrating the importance of
   networking?

❑ Can I find ways to improve the effectiveness of my team?

❑ Do I need to focus on remembering names?

❑ How do my listening skills impact my communication?

❑ Do I have a better understanding of gender differences in
   communication?

❑ Am I frequently apologizing when conversing with others?

❑ Am I doing all I can to enhance interdisciplinary
   communication?

❑ Have I considered getting a mentor?

❑ Am I courteous and respectful when dealing with colleagues?

❑ Can I identify gender differences in humor?

❑ Am I open and receptive to feedback?

Frequently Asked Questions

What is the best way to respond when colleagues get angry?

Don't take it personally. Try to focus on them and figure out their motivation. Why are they out of control? Put the blame on them—not on you (Shepard & Stimmler, 2005).

Do I need to play golf to advance my career?

No. If you're not comfortable playing golf, it won't help you. Any activity that you enjoy can help you connect with colleagues outside of the office.

How can I avoid office politics?

You can't. Office politics are inevitable and built into every job situation. Some call them corporate gamesmanship; others call them organization astuteness. You will be affected by office politics from day one in any job and in any industry (Klaus, 2007). Avoiding gossip and maintaining good relationships with your superiors and coworkers can ease the political climate for you.

Can you be your own mentor?

Yes. "You are your own best mentor. Know yourself and know what you need" (Evans, 2003, p. 74). You are responsible for your career. Coach yourself into taking the actions you need.

I am already overworked. How can I find more time to socialize with the team?

You are already part of the team. Prioritize your time so you don't overlook networking and mentoring opportunities. Having lunch with a colleague may do more to advance your career than an extra hour in the office (Evans, 2003).

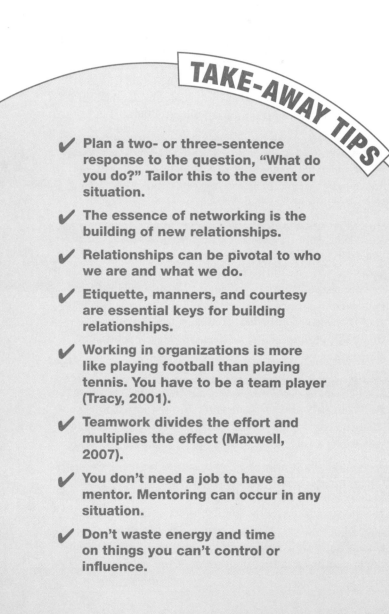

TAKE-AWAY TIPS

✓ Plan a two- or three-sentence response to the question, "What do you do?" Tailor this to the event or situation.

✓ The essence of networking is the building of new relationships.

✓ Relationships can be pivotal to who we are and what we do.

✓ Etiquette, manners, and courtesy are essential keys for building relationships.

✓ Working in organizations is more like playing football than playing tennis. You have to be a team player (Tracy, 2001).

✓ Teamwork divides the effort and multiplies the effect (Maxwell, 2007).

✓ You don't need a job to have a mentor. Mentoring can occur in any situation.

✓ Don't waste energy and time on things you can't control or influence.

2

✳

Developing Presentation Skills

The Planning Phase

Do you:

Avoid the biggest mistake speakers make when beginning a presentation?

Know the essential components of a strong beginning?

Consider your audience when planning a presentation?

Wonder how you can bring your content alive?

Know how to limit your content?

Public speaking is a powerful tool for informing, inspiring, persuading, and initiating action. As an integral tool of the business culture, presentations are an effective way to demonstrate leadership skills, gain recognition, and advance a career. Good presentation skills can leave an impression that a person can confidently and professionally demonstrate clear thinking and clear communication in a high-pressure situation. In essence, how you present yourself may be the difference between an upwardly mobile career and a dead-end job.

Few people can get up and present well off the top of their heads.
Preparation is the key to success.

*"One important key to success is self-confidence.
An important key to self-confidence is
preparation."*

—Arthur Ashe, Jr.

Planning for Success

Why is defining success a key component of preparation?

Having a purpose and defining success helps you set your goal for
the presentation. Your purpose must be clear in your mind so you
can relate it to your audience. For example, if your goal is to get five
volunteers for the health fair, you will know you succeeded if you
get at least five volunteers. If your goal is to motivate people to write
for the newsletter, you will know you succeeded when you see the
submissions. If your goal is to entertain the audience, laughter and
body language will support your success. As the adage goes, "If you
don't know where you're going, you'll probably end up somewhere
else."

Do you need a central theme?

Yes. A good speech needs a clearly identifiable theme. What do you
want your audience to know, think, or do after your presentation?
One way to think of this is to consider what audience members
would say afterwards if they were asked what the speech was about.
This is the main idea you want the audience to take home with
them. Decide what you want the word, phrase, or sentence to be,

then build your presentation to focus on this theme. For example, a group of childbirth educators used the theme of "preparation pays" for a very successful educational series for pregnant couples.

> *"Think as wise men do, but speak as the common people do."*
>
> —Aristotle

How to Begin

What is the best way to begin a presentation?

You should grab the audience's attention with something compelling like a story, a question, or a quote. As Doug Stevenson (2009) says, "Just because peoples' butts are in the seats, doesn't mean their brains are in the room." When you face an audience, you may be looking at people preoccupied by many things. For example, they may be thinking about the presentation that preceded yours, the work piling up in their office, or a conversation they just had (Steele, 2009).

You need a "grabber" or attention getter. Here are some examples:

* Current events
* Unusual facts
* Questions
* Statistics
* Quotes
* Stories or examples
* Comparisons and contrasts

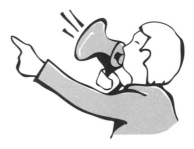

What is the biggest mistake a presenter makes when beginning a presentation?

Some presenters have the tendency to begin weak and try to build up to a strong presentation. They can immediately improve their presentations if they begin strong with a grabber, as mentioned previously. Here are some things not to say or do at the beginning of a presentation:

* "Today, I'm going to talk about . . ."

* "I know this is boring, but . . . "

* "I am sorry I am not as prepared . . ."

* "I don't know why I was asked to speak on this topic, but . . . "

* "I won't take up too much of your time."

* "So, how is everybody doing?"

* "Please bear with me. I'm really nervous."

* "Let's review some housekeeping details . . . "

* "I'm getting over the flu and . . . "

* Don't share personal experiences unless they relate to the topic.

* Avoid overworked quotations.

* Avoid dictionary definitions because they are boring and condescending.

(Brody, 2008; Lindsell-Roberts, 2000)

Communication Coach

Tammy had planned to show a video clip as part of her presentation. During her presentation, she spent a lot of time trying unsuccessfully to get the clip to run. She apologized to the audience numerous times during her presentation.

Lesson: It is not in the speaker's best interest to keep reminding the audience what they are not getting. Repeated apologies are distracting.

How can you get the audience to "buy into" your topic?

You must be able to answer the question "What's in it for them (WIIFT)?" People will not be interested if the topic does not pertain to them. You must tell them why this presentation is worth their time and how it can help them. For example, years ago I was the guest speaker for a middle school English class. I was asked to speak about how I wrote my first book. The students did not seem too interested until I asked them what questions they had. One brave boy raised his hand and asked if I made money writing. When I said, "Yes, I make a lot of money," I suddenly had their interest and enthusiasm. I was now addressing WIIFT with a lively audience.

Do you have any suggestions for incorporating WIIFY (What's in it for you)?

Yes. Here are some suggestions:

* ❋ "This is important to you because . . . "

* ❋ "So, you may be wondering what this means to you."

* ❋ "You may be thinking, 'Who cares?' You should care because . . . "

* ❋ "Why am I telling you this?"

(Weissman, 2005)

How do you establish credibility as a speaker?

This is vital to answering the question "Why should we listen to you?" There are several ways to do this, such as mentioning your education, experience, research, publications, and so on. This should be part of your introduction and should relate to the topic of the presentation. For example, if you are speaking about orthopedic nursing, describe your education, position, and experience in this clinical area. If someone does not introduce you, you must introduce yourself and establish your credibility. You could say, "Good morning. I'm . . ." and then establish your credibility.

Should you provide an overview when you begin your presentation?

Yes. This helps the audience follow along. It may also keep them from shuffling through a handout to find this information. Take note as you watch the television news. The host will always give an overview of the show. This is meant to entice you to keep watching. You want to achieve the same goal with your overview.

Targeting the Audience

How can you best connect with the audience?

Remember that your presentation is for the audience, not for you. Put yourself in their shoes. How can you address their needs and their goals? What would be meaningful to them? The best speeches make a connection between the speaker and the audience.

BAKER COLLEGE OF
CLINTON TWP. LIBRAR'

Communication Coach

Marjorie was asked to keynote a church banquet for senior citizens. She began with a heartwarming story about a 100-year-old patient and explained how this story's lesson could apply to them. Because many of the men had served in the military, she related a story from her days as an Army nurse.

Lesson: She endeared herself to the audience by gearing the presentation to their interests and experiences.

What do you need to know about your audience?

The more you learn about them, the better you relate to them. You can also avoid offending anyone and including too much or too little information. Here are some things to consider:

* What are the demographics (age, sex, education, race, income, occupation) of the audience?

* Why are they attending your presentation? Do they want to attend or do they have to?

* How much do they know about the subject matter?

* Does the audience have any particular issues or concerns?

* What will they take away to make their jobs or lives better?

* Will they view you as a credible presenter?

(Lindsell-Roberts, 2000)

How can you find out information about the audience?

A good source for audience information will be the program organizer. You can also use the Internet, newsletters, annual reports, and promotional materials to help you learn more about the group. The time it takes to prepare an audience profile could make the difference between success and failure. For example, imagine how upset you would be if you begin your speech discussing a new method of birth control to a group of retired war veterans (Brody, 2008).

Body of the Presentation

What are the key elements of the body of a presentation?

The body should progress logically, be easy to follow, and emphasize major points. Its content should keep the audience involved.

Why should you use transitions?

Remember, you are not doing the presentation for yourself but for the audience. Transitions are helpful for the audience. They provide a guidepost for where you are going. For example, suppose you want to transition from talking about drug indications to drug administration. Try this, "Now that we've talked about the indications for this new drug, how is it administered?" Transitions are so much more effective than saying, "Next slide please." Using transitions greatly improves your presentations, so plan your transitions before giving the presentation.

You can observe good transitions while watching TV talk or news shows. For example, "When we return after a break, we'll have Dennis Miller giving his opinion about the . . . " People like to know what is coming next. When you are giving a presentation, you are the only who knows where you are going unless you supply transitions.

How can you bring your content alive?

The key here is to have variety. Use the grabbers previously mentioned. Keep the attention of the audience by incorporating comparisons, metaphors, similes, alliteration, and analogies. For example, you could use this analogy when discussing electroencephalograms

(EEG) with a non-medical audience: "An ECG is to the heart as an EEG is to the brain. Both detect electrical activity."

How can you avoid a data dump?

You must avoid information overload. Keep your content alive and relevant. Audience members can only accept so much information without a chance to process the information by discussion, analysis, questioning, or taking a break. As a colleague of mine says, "Don't just show up and throw up."

Never go over your time. This is inconsiderate to your audience. A speaker needs to end on time regardless of what time he or she started.

How can you avoid having too much information?

Use the 75% rule. If you have 60 minutes for a presentation, plan for 45 minutes. Divide your material into must-know, should-know, and could-know (Brody, 2008) categories, and perhaps color code this material. If you are running out of time, focus on the must-know and eliminate the others as needed.

Focusing on the must-know content was invaluable for me several years ago when I was doing a business etiquette luncheon program for 150 people. I was supposed to speak from 12:30 PM to 1:30 PM. The group arrived late after getting a group photo and had to go through a buffet line. I was not able to start my presentation until 1:03 PM, yet I ended at 1:29 PM. The conference planner was impressed and appreciative.

"The more you say, the less people remember."

–Anatole France

Telling Stories

Do you have any suggestions for stories?

Yes, the story must relate to the topic and/or illustrate a key point in your presentation. According to William Steele, when a speaker transitions to a story or example, the audience senses that something is being brought to life to help make the message more real or understandable. Audiences love to hear, "Let me give you an example" (Steele, 2009). They perk up and listen.

Stephen Denning found that audiences "co-create" stories by adding to the story with their own mental pictures of the settings and the participants. He said this explains why the only things some people can remember weeks after a presentation are the stories the speaker told (Denning, 2001). Stories separate a good speaker from a great speaker and a dry presentation from an interesting one.

How can you be sure your story is appropriate for the audience?

Use your audience assessment as a guide. For example, don't tell stories about your children at an infertility conference. Avoid telling jokes that make fun of anyone other than you. Someone in the group may have a problem (such as obesity) or be sympathetic to someone you make fun of (Brody, 2008).

TIP

To write an effective speech, replace the rules for written English with the rules for spoken, conversational English.

What is a good length for a story?

Stories or anecdotes should be short accounts of an interesting incident. Steele recommends thinking of a story as a slide-length component of your message. The time you take to tell the story should be about the same as the time you would spend on one of your slides (Steele, 2009).

Do stories have to be funny?

No. Stories can arouse empathy, create surprise, provide inspiration, emphasize key points, or even agitate people so that they take action.

Communication Coach

Greg attended a presentation given by a renowned world scientist. He was very disappointed listening to the professor read his entire presentation. Most everyone had left the room by the time the presentation was finished. Several weeks later, the same findings were published and received great feedback.

Lesson: An effective speech needs to be different from a written paper.

Incorporating Humor

Do you need to be funny to be a good presenter?

No. But, without a doubt, humor certainly helps in a presentation. However, some people are not good at being funny, and they should not try to be funny if that is not their forte. If you do say something intended to be humorous, don't smile or laugh unless the audience reacts first with smiles or laughter. If nobody laughs or smiles, just keep moving along without leaving the impression that something has fallen flat (Steele, 2009).

Are telling jokes the main way to add humor?

No, you do not need to tell jokes to provide humor. Instead of aiming for laughter, aim for smiles. The safest humor revolves around stories about you. The story can liven up your message without having the audience rolling in the aisles with laughter. They may be smiling and nodding while enjoying the story. Your story doesn't need a punch line and it has validity by being something you experienced (Steele, 2009).

What's a good way to start incorporating humor into a presentation?

Cartoons are great options. You can simply describe a cartoon or you can show a cartoon on a slide (if you have permission). Practice this and other forms of humor with your friends and family. If you get a good response, use it in a presentation.

How to Close With Impact

How important is the ending of a presentation?

The end is as important as the beginning. People tend to remember what they heard first and last. The ending must be strong. Poor endings are a result of neglect. By mistake, some presenters think the presentation ends after the last question.

The ending gives the presenter time to restate the purpose, review key points, and end with something memorable. For example, the presenter can say, "If you only remember one thing . . . " or "My main take-away is . . . " A strong ending may be a call for action that the audience needs to take.

Are there things not to say or do at the end of a presentation?

Yes, to end with impact, avoid saying or doing the following:

 * "I'm sorry this was boring . . . "

 * "I forgot to mention . . . "

* Introducing a new idea or new research study.

* Going over your time allotment.

* Packing your materials while you are talking.

* Answering the last question and not using a planned ending.

TIP

While using PowerPoint, press the "B" key on your computer's keyboard to blank or blacken the screen. It will stay that way until you press the "B" key again. Do this when you want the audience to look at you instead of the screen. This is effective during your opening and closing and also during breaks between slides.

✗ The Cardinal Sins of Presentations

No clear point: The audience leaves the session thinking, "What was the point?"

No audience benefit: The audience members think, "So what?"

No clear flow: The audience is confused and cannot follow the presentation.

Too detailed: The main point was obscured by numerous or irrelevant facts.

Too long: The audience gets bored and loses focus before the presentation ends.

(Weissman, 2005)

Using Visuals

Why are visuals important in a presentation?

They keep the attention of the audience and add interest. They should reinforce and illustrate the message. I want to emphasize that a good visual does not make up for a poor presentation. Don't expect your visuals to carry you through a poorly planned presentation. Most presentations use PowerPoint slides.

What are some tips for improving PowerPoint slides?

Here are some tips to improve your presentations.

* Craft your message before you make your slides to prevent fragmented pieces of information (Steele, 2009).

* Make your visuals for the audience. They are not notes for the speaker. They should help the audience follow and understand your message.

* Don't put too much information on a slide.

* If you need a good handout, know that a slide show is not a good handout.

* Don't have a slide showing all the time. A blank screen directs the attention back to you. Try this at the beginning and end of your presentation (Brody, 2008).

* Be visual with visuals. Remember a picture is worth a thousand words. But, don't use a visual or image if it does not contribute to your message.

* Replace long sentences and paragraphs with bulleted phrases.

* Choose a typeface that is easy to read. Sans-serif is ideal for headlines and serif is better for text. (Serif refers to the small line finishing off the stroke of a letter.) Be consistent and use the same font for all titles and text. Use a minimum of 18- to

22-point type (Brody, 2008). Use upper and lower case letters.

* Don't read your slides. This is patronizing to the audience (Weissman, 2004).

* Navigate the slide deck smoothly. Learn to jump around without running through intervening slides. When using PowerPoint, you can jump to another slide by typing the slide number on your computer and pressing the "enter" key. Keep a numbered list of your slides next to your laptop. You can print a list of slides by collapsing the outline of your presentation to titles and hitting the "print" command.

✔ Checklist

Pre-Presentation Preparation

- ❑ Did I define success for this presentation?
- ❑ Is my central theme clear?
- ❑ Did I research and target the audience?
- ❑ Do I begin with an attention getter?
- ❑ Do I answer the question WIIFT (what's in it for them)?
- ❑ Is my credibility established?
- ❑ Does my opening include an overview?
- ❑ Have I planned out my transitions?
- ❑ Do my visuals support my content?
- ❑ Did I follow the 75% rule?
- ❑ Did I bring the content alive with examples, stories, humor, etc?
- ❑ Am I ending with impact?

Frequently Asked Questions

 Doesn't all this planning get in the way of sounding spontaneous?

No. The spontaneity you want comes after planning and preparation. After you carefully craft a presentation and practice it, you can then sound spontaneous. As Peter Hall, the former director of England's National Theatre says, "You have to have the discipline and then you will be liberated by it" (Steele, 2009).

 What is the best way to find stories for your presentations?

Collect stories. When you experience something or hear about something that might make a good anecdote in a future presentation, write it down. You can get ideas from watching TV, listening to the radio, reading, talking to people, and being more observant of things happening in your daily life. Think back in your life to meaningful events or situations that would provide a good story or example. Keep a file of stories.

 How can you avoid offending people with jokes?

Be careful. Many people are looking for a possible offense. Political correctness is a minefield. Sometimes, knowing in advance whether a joke is safe can be difficult. If you have any question about offending someone in the audience or someone they know, avoid the joke. There are other ways to be funny without telling jokes.

How do you avoid being perceived as self-centered when you tell stories?

Don't make yourself the hero or heroine of your stories or anecdotes. Tell something amusing, strange, or enlightening that happened to a friend, neighbor, family member, co-worker, or acquaintance.

 Suppose you are getting near the end of your presentation and you think you will not have time for a great story. What should you do?

Skip the story to avoid going over your time. The audience doesn't need to know that you are skipping something. They would rather end early than end late. Who hasn't appreciated getting out early from a presentation? Ending 5 minutes early is better than ending 2 minutes late.

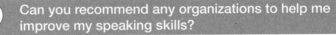 **Can you recommend any organizations to help me improve my speaking skills?**

Yes. Join Toastmasters, the international organization made up of thousands of local clubs. You can practice speaking and receive peer review. Visit www.toastmasters.org to find out more. For advanced speakers, I recommend visiting www.nsaspeaker. org for tips from the National Speakers Association.

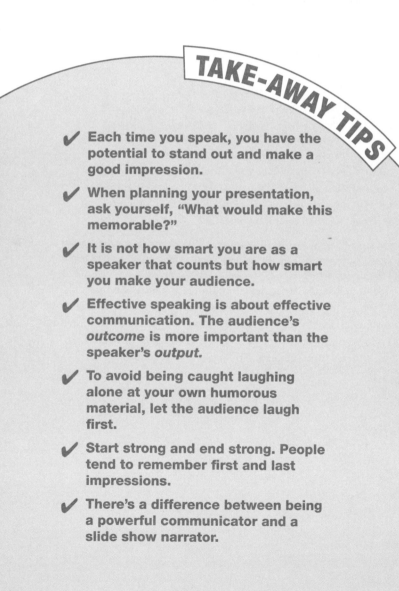

TAKE-AWAY TIPS

✔ Each time you speak, you have the potential to stand out and make a good impression.

✔ When planning your presentation, ask yourself, "What would make this memorable?"

✔ It is not how smart you are as a speaker that counts but how smart you make your audience.

✔ Effective speaking is about effective communication. The audience's *outcome* is more important than the speaker's *output.*

✔ To avoid being caught laughing alone at your own humorous material, let the audience laugh first.

✔ Start strong and end strong. People tend to remember first and last impressions.

✔ There's a difference between being a powerful communicator and a slide show narrator.

3

＊

Developing Presentation Skills

Practice and Delivery

Do you:

Know the best ways to practice for your presentation?

Wonder how you can get good feedback during your practice sessions?

Consider the visual, vocal, and verbal components of communication?

Know how to manage fear, anxiety, and jitters?

Navigate PowerPoint with finesse?

Use the ABC method for handling questions?

Some people think that once they have planned their presentation, the hard work is over. This is a mistake. An effective presentation requires a significant time commitment for practice. Although great speakers make it look easy, you will be shocked when you learn how much time they spend practicing. This chapter describes the behind-the-scenes strategies of effective speakers for practice and delivery of great presentations.

"We are what we repeatedly do. Excellence is therefore not an act but a habit."

—Aristotle

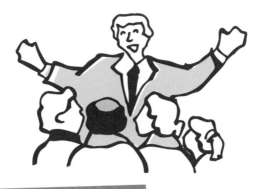

How to Practice

What are some effective strategies for practicing before a presentation?

Practice out loud. Don't look over your notes and say, "blah, blah, blah." Many of us are eloquent in our heads. There is a world of difference between ideas in your head and speaking to an audience. When you practice out loud, you will hear when you stumble over words or hesitate because you are unsure of something. This alerts you to the need to make changes.

Focus on the visual, vocal, and verbal aspects of your communication. The professional impression we make is based on the words we use (verbal), the way our voices sound (vocal), and what people see (visual). Words alone have a small impact on effective communication. The visual and vocal elements have a stronger impact. So, consider this when you practice. Your dress, grooming, and body language will impact your presentation along with the sound of your voice. For example, if you say you are happy to be somewhere, but you are looking at your watch and you sound bored, the audience will not believe your words.

Some experts say you will be more successful with a well-practiced "B" level presentation than a "Grade A" presentation that was not adequately rehearsed (Steele, 2009).

"The mind is more slowly stirred by the ear than by the eye."

–Homer

How do you know when you have practiced enough?

I have found that after a certain point of practice, I "cross the line." For me, this means that I am so well prepared that I would be very disappointed if the program were cancelled.

Dale Carnegie, the speech guru, said that there are three speeches for every one you actually give. These are the speech you practiced, the speech you gave, and the speech you wish you had given. Only through practice can all three potentially be the same.

Communication Coach

One of my favorite *The Far Side* cartoons by Gary Larson is about Tarzan as he prepares to meet Jane. In his head, he eloquently prepares several nice introductory remarks. However, when he swings on a vine and lands near her in a tree, he blurts out, "Me Tarzan! You Jane!" Then, he swears and covers his face with his hands.

Lesson: Your ideas can flow beautifully and eloquently in your mind. Practice out loud.

"Let our advance worrying become advance thinking and planning."

–Sir Winston Churchill

Managing Fear, Anxiety, and Jitters

How do you handle fear, anxiety, and jitters?

All speakers feel this way. The key is to handle these feelings in a productive manner. Think of fear as your friend to increase your energy level, add a little color to your cheeks, and put a sparkle in your eyes. Think of nervousness as "performance energy" to prevent a bland and boring presentation. Fear also makes you want to practice and prepare. Use fear to your benefit. The more you practice, the less fear, anxiety, and jitters you will have.

Turn the focus away from you. Don't think about yourself. Think about the audience. Remember the audience is not there to judge you. They are there to learn something and you are prepared to provide it (Gottesman & Buzz, 2001).

TIP

Focus not on how smart you are as the speaker, but on how smart you can make your audience.

Have a positive attitude. View your upcoming presentation as an opportunity for success instead of a potential for failure. Visualize yourself as confident and doing a great job.

What can I do to relieve stress before the presentation?

Visit the room where you will be speaking. Walk to the front and visualize how the room will be set up.

Get a good night's sleep. Eat your usual meals. If you normally exercise, do that to help reduce your stress. Do some abdominal breathing. Rolling your head, yawning, and making funny faces also help to reduce stress.

Get to the presentation site early and mingle with some members of the audience. Ask them questions and listen carefully to their answers. Try to gather information and names you can incorporate into your presentation (Weissman, 2004).

Avoid negative thoughts and negative people. Think positive. Make affirming statements (Detz, 2000). For example, "I really know this material . . . I have been preparing this for months . . . I have a lot of helpful information to share."

How can you handle stress during the presentation?

Never say, "I'm really nervous." This is upsetting to the audience and makes them uncomfortable. Focus on the audience. Intensify your eye contact. Change the dynamics. For example, you could ask a question or ask the audience members to discuss something with the person next to them. Another technique is to invite the audience to share reactions, stories, or ideas.

How can you handle a dry mouth?

Plan ahead and have water available. If you do not have any, try gently biting the tip of your tongue. This helps you to salivate. You can also lightly coat your teeth with petroleum jelly to stop your lips from sticking to your teeth (Brody, 2008).

"Fear is a big factor in diving. It's a part of the sport; it's a part of overcoming the sport; it's a part of the thrill of the sport."

—Michele Mitchell-Rocha

Communication Coach

Whenever Winston Churchill delivered a speech, he always had notes with him. However, he seldom used them. When asked about this, Churchill replied, "I carry fire insurance, but I don't expect my house to burn down" (Chaney & Martin, 2007).

Lesson: Bring and use your notes as necessary.

Getting Feedback

How can I get feedback before my presentation?

The best way is to videotape yourself to critique what you see and hear. Try to be objective and critical while you listen to and observe your presentation. Do you have distracting gestures? Are you stumbling over certain words or phrases? Are you using fillers (ah, um, like, you know)? Replace them with a pause. Focus on making these improvements. Then practice and videotape again. This process will keep improving your presentation.

What if I cannot videotape myself?

The next best thing is to audiotape yourself. Although you will miss out on the visual components, you will still be able to evaluate the vocal and verbal aspects of the presentation. Keep repeating this process until you sound competent and confident.

How about getting a peer to evaluate your presentation?

This is a great idea. Ask the person to provide several tips to improve the presentation. Ask if the person noted any distracting gestures. Ask what sections were unclear?

How about evaluation forms?

These are great for feedback after your presentation. Most speakers focus on their weaknesses. We can surely learn from them. But we also learn from our strengths. Keep your evaluations short. See the following list for some ideas for an evaluation form.

Post Presentation Evaluation

Please help me evaluate and improve this program. Your constructive criticism would be greatly appreciated.

- What did you like most about this program?

- What did you like least about this program?

- What is the best idea you got from this program?

- What can the speaker do to improve?

- Please rate the following on a scale of 1 (worst) to 10 (best). Please circle your choice.

    - Content: (worst) 1 2 3 4 5 6 7 8 9 10 (best)

    - Delivery: (worst) 1 2 3 4 5 6 7 8 9 10 (best)

Thank you for taking the time to evaluate my presentation.
K. D. Pagana

Using Flip Charts

When can you use flip charts?

Flip charts are good for small, informal groups. They can also be a welcome relief from back-to-back PowerPoint programs. You can write points as you speak or put your points on the charts before the meeting. You can tear off the sheets and post them around the room.

Are there any guidelines for using flip charts?

Yes. Here are some basic points to follow:

* Use large letters (2 to 4 inches high). The larger the audience, the larger the lettering that is needed.

* Use upper and lower case letters.

* Black or blue markers are easiest to read.

* Avoid red and green markers together because many people are color-blind.

* Follow the 4 x 4 rule: use no more than 4 lines and no more than 4 words per line.

* Write only on the upper three-fourths of the paper because the audience will have difficulty seeing below this point.

* Some presenters print their points lightly in pencil on the paper prior to their presentation. Then, during the presentation, they write over the points with a marker.

TIP

Apply the three Ts (touch, turn, and talk) while you use your visual aids. After you touch the key point, turn to the audience, establish eye contact, and then continue to talk (Brody, 2008).

(Brody, 2008)

Using White Boards

When can you use white boards?

The dry-erase white board is the descendent of the traditional black board. Both can be effective in smaller groups. Many of the principles discussed with flip charts also apply.

White boards work well for impromptu sessions when the presenter can write one point on the board at a time and then discuss it. They also work for viewing a large amount of detail. In this case, the content can be drawn on the white board before the audience arrives (Yate & Sander, 2003).

Be sure to avoid using permanent markers in place of the dry-erase markers.

Using PowerPoint

How can I navigate PowerPoint with finesse?

Navigating slides with finesse takes a lot of practice. Remember that PowerPoint slides should support your presentation. They are not the key element. Here are some tips to improve your PowerPoint presentations:

* Talk to the audience, not the slide. Don't turn your back on the audience.

* If you are standing to the side of the screen, stand on the left side. People read from left to right.

* Don't read the slides. Slides should supplement what you say, not repeat it.

* Never block the light source of the projector when you gesture or move.

* Answer the "so what?" Give the audience time to become familiar with the slide. Remember you have seen the slide many times, but this is the first time for the audience. Clarify the slide if it is complex.

* Plan your transitions. To hear a speaker keep saying, "The next slide shows . . . " is boring for an audience. Instead, transition from one slide to another. For example, suppose your current slide is about drug indications and the next one is about side effects. Before moving to the new slide, say something like, "Now that we've discussed drug indications, you may be wondering about side effects." Jot down your transitions on photocopies of the slides (Steele, 2009).

* Make use of the "B" key. This blanks or blackens the screen and directs the attention back to you. Only keep a slide on the screen when you are discussing its content. For example, if someone asks a question, blacken the screen. This makes the audience look at you instead of staring at the screen. This is especially important to use at the beginning and end of your presentation.

* Jump around the slides without annoying the audience. When using PowerPoint, just type the slide number and hit the "enter" key to move to any slide in your presentation. This is very helpful if you are running out of time and want to skip a few slides. This technique is invaluable if someone asks a question and you want to reference a slide you used earlier.

* Remember Murphy's Law. You never know what may happen, so be prepared to do the presentation without the PowerPoint slides. This is preferable to becoming flustered and wasting a lot of time. Print and bring a hard copy of your presentation.

* Back-up your slides. Bring a copy of your program on a thumb drive or memory stick for possible transfer to another laptop. Additionally, e-mail yourself a copy of your presentation so you could go online and download your program if necessary.

Communication Coach

Monika was leading a continuing education seminar on Appreciative Inquiry. She was using a PowerPoint slide show and a DVD. During the DVD, she kept the PowerPoint slide showing the entire time. This detracted from the impact of the DVD. After her presentation, a more experienced faculty member showed Monika how to utilize the "B" key and black out the screen.

Lesson: When you are not using the PowerPoint slide, black out the screen by using the "B" key.

Setting the Tone

Who determines the tone of your presentation?

You do. No matter what kind of vibes you are getting from the audience, you must set the tone. Establish an upbeat tone and stick with it. Most audiences will eventually come around and respond to this positive atmosphere (Steele, 2009).

What are some things to avoid when trying to set the tone?

Speakers should not chide the audience. As an audience member, I find it annoying when a speaker says, "Good morning" and then criticizes the audience's weak response and makes them keep repeating the phrase louder each time. That sets a bad tone for connecting with the audience.

Breathing Time

When should you give the audience breathing time?

Sometimes when you are delivering a heavy message, the audience may feel overwhelmed and need a break. For example, you have probably seen this demonstrated when someone is delivering a eulogy. The speaker knows to lighten up at times and say something humorous. This gives the audience a needed chance to catch their breath. If you don't provide breathing time, the audience may need to tune you out to find some relief (Steele, 2009).

Are there other ways to lighten up besides using humor?

Yes. For example, if you were discussing a tragic accident, you could give the audience some relief by complimenting the emergency care and the nursing staff. You could also describe some procedural issue related to your topic. Breathing time shows your sensitivity to the potentially suffocating nature of some messages.

Ending on Time

If you are giving a great presentation, is it really important to end on time?

Yes, if you respect your audience. Going over your time limit leads to one of the biggest audience complaints. If you start and end on time, you will score points with your audience. You will also get better audience participation. It is unlikely that anyone would want to ask a question if you are over your time limit. (Steele, 2009).

Remember, you can jump slides if you are running out of time. Also, you can cut material by focusing on "must-know" versus "could-know" content.

What if factors beyond your control create the likelihood of running late?

Talk to your audience and see what they are interested in doing. Be willing to stop at the end time and make arrangements for them to get the remaining information by other means. For example, they could send you an e-mail or go to a link on your website. If most want you to stay late and continue, that is also okay. Be sure to give permission for others to leave at any time.

Platform Skills and Tips

Are there any specific skills or tips to improve your effectiveness on the platform?

Yes, there are a number of things you can do. I recommend focusing on one or two at a time. After mastering the first few you pick, add another one or two. You will find that your presentation skills improve after every presentation. Here are some suggestions (Steele, 2009):

* **Own the geography.** Don't stand in one place. Move around, but move with purpose. Don't overdo it. Be sure to make eye contact with everyone. Use a remote control so you can advance your slides without staying behind a podium or being chained to your laptop.

* **Use good eye contact.** When you finish a presentation, everyone in the room should feel like you spoke to him or her. Don't stare. This can be interpreted as aggression or affection. You don't want a fight and you don't want a date. Your goal is to connect with the audience members.

* **Develop an effective speaking voice.** Use variety in your volume, tone, and animation. People tire of listening to weak voices. If you speak in a clear, loud, and animated tone, you will sound more confident. People will take notice and listen.

Many speakers could dramatically improve with some voice lessons.

* **Sound like you care.** If you want your audience to care about something, you have to sound like you care. They need to hear in your voice that you care.

* **Pause for effect.** A pause emphasizes the last thing you said and gives it a chance to sink in with your audience. A pause can also signal a change in direction or thought. Think of reading a book. Without any pauses, a book would be exhausting to read or hear read aloud. A presentation without pauses would have that same quality. Strong speakers use pauses. When you practice, practice the pauses.

* **Use appropriate gestures.** A good idea is to videotape a presentation and review it on fast forward. Your movements will be exaggerated and you can see whether your gestures are distracting. The best way to add some variety to your gestures is to do some rough pantomiming. For example, if you are talking about a large textbook, show the size and thickness with your hands. See the following list for the keys to effective gesturing (Brody, 2008).

  * Use gestures to emphasize your main points.
  * Vary your gestures.
  * Don't point at your audience with your finger or fist.
  * Keep your palms open to your audience.
  * Gesture using your arm and hand together as a single unit.

TIP

Volunteer to give a presentation. This will give you a great opportunity to prepare, practice, present, and get feedback. Your volunteerism will also be noticed and appreciated.

* Use large gestures for a large audience and small gestures for a small audience.
* Don't cross your arms in front of you or behind your back.
* Keep your hands out of your pockets.
* Keep your gestures above your waist.
* Smiling makes you seem confident.

Impromptu Speaking

What is impromptu speaking?

Impromptu speaking is often referred to as off-the-cuff speaking. You speak on the spur of the moment with minimal time to prepare your remarks. The impromptu style is best suited to casual remarks that only last a few minutes (Gottesman & Buzz, 2001). For example, at a meeting, you may be asked to comment about something or give an opinion.

Is there a way to be successful with impromptu speaking?

Yes. Try to anticipate whether you may be asked to speak and come prepared, just in case. Feel free to pause for a few seconds to collect your thoughts. No one expects you to start speaking immediately.

Rather than mumbling, talking in circles, or apologizing for not being prepared, many people have benefited by using the PREP technique (Brody, 2008) in impromptu situations. After pausing, here is the guide for your response:

✳ **P**oint of view/position/opinion: "My point of view . . . " or
"In my opinion . . . "

✳ **R**eason: "The reason is . . . "

✳ **E**xample/explanation: "As an example . . . "

✳ **P**oint of view: "Therefore, my point of view is . . . "

For example, suppose I am asked for my opinion about the various options for the office renovations. A response using the PREP technique could be, "From my point of view, the second option is the best. The reason is that we need more conference room space. For example, it takes several weeks to book the conference room. Therefore, according to my point of view, I would recommend the second option." Using the PREP model helps you sound logical and concise. People may be impressed with how succinct you are when put on the spot.

"It usually takes me more than three weeks to write a good impromptu speech."

–Mark Twain

Handling Q & A

Do you have any suggestions for handling questions and answers?

Yes. Early in your presentation, tell the audience when you will be taking questions. You could save them for the end, take them at specific breaking points, or take them throughout the presentation.

Give the audience time to ask questions. Look at the audience. (Some speakers ask about questions and then look at their notes and can't see the raised hand.) Encourage questions by having an open body stance and enthusiasm.

Use the ABC approach.

* **A**nticipate: Try to anticipate what may be asked. Write down the questions you are asked because you will probably get them again in the future. The next time you will be prepared.

* Be **B**rief: Answer the question briefly without a lot of background information. If you take a long time to answer, people won't want to ask other questions.

* Keep **C**ontrol: You need to remain in control of the topic and the audience. If the questions take you off topic, get back on track. Don't let any person dominate the Q & A session.

Who should the speaker look at when someone in the audience asks a question?

You should begin and end answering the question by looking at the questioner. But, during the answer, you should also give eye contact to other people in the audience. This keeps you connected to the whole audience (Steele, 2009).

How can you get the Q & A session started?

Don't do what speakers typically do, saying, "Does anyone have a question?" Many people do not respond because this implies that they need help understanding the material (Steele, 2009). Instead, say, "Who has the first question?" or "What questions do you have?" This implies that questions are expected, and you are asking who is going to start.

A great tip is to prepare a stimulating question or two to get the questions started. For example, say, "One question I am often asked is . . . " Having this question planned ahead of time is a great way to get the questions started. Once you get the ball rolling, the audience will be more likely to pick it up and run with it (Gottesman &

Mauro, 2001). Your starting question is also a great way to address something you may have forgotten to include in the presentation.

What can you do about someone who dominates the Q & A session?

This person is a stage hog. Stage hogs demand attention and want everyone to look at them and listen to them. If unrestrained, they will derail your presentation. You need to act early and discourage this unproductive competition.

After the person asks several questions, say, "Thanks for your questions, but I want to give others a chance as well. I would be happy to speak more with you after the session." If this doesn't work, make the stage hog feel responsible for delaying others in the audience. For example, "We are supposed to end at 4 p.m. Is it okay with the rest of you to move on so we can end on time?"

What if someone asks a question and you do not know the answer?

Be honest. Here are several options:

* Ask whether someone else knows the answer.

* Say you do not know, but that you will get back to the person with the answer. Write the question down and ask the person to provide contact information before leaving.

* If you know where the information can be found, tell them. For example, "I don't know the answer, but I know it is on the American Cancer Society website."

If there is an expert in the room who could answer a question, should you refer to him or her?

It would be polite to ask the expert before the presentation whether he or she would be willing to help with the Q & A. Later, if you want to ask the expert to answer a question, be sure to repeat the question in case the expert was not paying attention and missed the question.

 Checklist

Practicing Your Presentation

❑ Did I allow sufficient time to practice?

❑ Did I practice out loud?

❑ Did I use the normal nervousness associated with a presentation to my benefit?

❑ Did I videotape or audiotape myself for feedback? Did I prepare an evaluation form?

❑ Did I practice navigating through my PowerPoint program?

❑ Do I know how to use the "B" key and how to jump slides?

❑ Have I prepared a back-up plan in case of equipment failure?

❑ Did I practice using gestures and pauses?

❑ Do I have a commonly asked question to use to start the Q & A session?

Frequently Asked Questions

If you start your PowerPoint presentation without a slide, when do you show your title slide?

Show the title slide while the audience is entering the room and getting settled. Then, blank the screen and concentrate on making eye contact with the audience before beginning your presentation.

Is it okay to end the presentation with the last question?

No. You will lose control of the ending if you do. You should end with your memorable statement. Think of what you want the audience to walk out of the room thinking about. End with that. For example, if the last question is related to validating a parking pass and you end there, people might be thinking about parking passes on the way out of the room. Instead, try to end with control and impact, such as, "If you only remember one thing, please remember . . . "

 When practicing, should you try to memorize your presentation?

You do not need to memorize the script. Stay flexible in your word use and say things differently with each practice so you don't sound rehearsed. Practicing helps smooth your rough spots (Steele, 2009).

 Should you always repeat the question during a Q & A session?

Either repeat the question or answer in a full sentence. For example, if someone asks about the normal dose of Evista, you can repeat the question and give the answer or say, "The normal dose of Evista is 60 mg orally once a day."

How do you handle eye contact with a large audience?

Look toward groups of people. This will give the impression of eye contact to individual members of the group.

What can you do if you get red splotches on your face and neck when speaking?

Wear pink or red colors with high necklines. The red splotches will not be as noticeable in comparison to when you wear white.

How do you handle shaky legs or knocking knees?

Walk around or shift your weight from one leg to another.

 I often hear speakers begin to answer a question by saying, "That's a good question." What do you think?

Avoid that phrase because it makes it seem like you are grading the questions. Also, if you compliment one questioner, it is awkward if you don't compliment the others. A better way to foster a positive relationship with the audience is to preface your response with, "I appreciate your question," or "That is a concern for many of us" (Gottesman & Buzz, 2001).

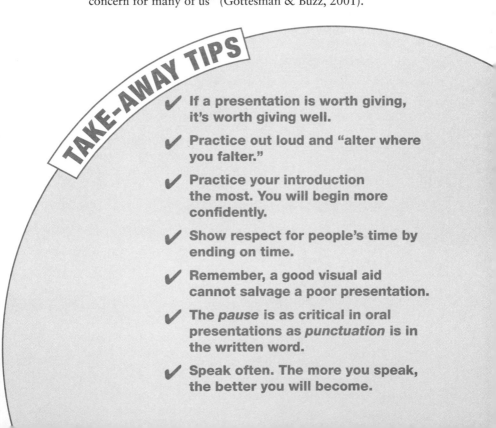

TAKE-AWAY TIPS

✔ **If a presentation is worth giving, it's worth giving well.**

✔ **Practice out loud and "alter where you falter."**

✔ **Practice your introduction the most. You will begin more confidently.**

✔ **Show respect for people's time by ending on time.**

✔ **Remember, a good visual aid cannot salvage a poor presentation.**

✔ **The *pause* is as critical in oral presentations as *punctuation* is in the written word.**

✔ **Speak often. The more you speak, the better you will become.**

4

*

Writing Business Letters, Memos, Reports, and Notes

Do you:

Ever read a letter, memo, or message and struggle to get the point of it?

Write clearly and concisely?

Consider the visual impact of your message?

Have the right tone for your message?

Know the key components of a business letter and memo?

Organize your thoughts to have the most effect on your reader?

Exceptional writing is a distinguishing characteristic of exceptional professionals. A well-written message may gain you recognition, bolster your reputation, or influence decisions. Writing, like any skill, can be improved by knowing the basics and practicing. Although the methods of writing have changed from quill pens to typewriters to computers, one thing has not changed—the need to get your point across in a clear and concise manner (Lindsell-Roberts, 2004).

"I hope you will pardon me for writing such a long letter, but I did not have time to write you a shorter one."

–Blaise Pascal

Writing Guidelines

Does your written communication influence your professional impact?

Most definitely. First impressions are difficult to change, including impressions formed because of your written communication. Messages with inconsistent formatting, poor writing style, or incorrect punctuation and grammar create a poor impression. Sloppy writing leads the receiver to think that the quality of the writer, and the services of the company, may be inferior (Chaney & Martin, 2007).

Do you have any suggestions to make business messages more effective?

Here are some guidelines to follow:

* Write clearly and concisely. Avoid unnecessary words. For example, rather than saying, "At this point in time," say, "Now." See Table 4.1 for windbag phrases to avoid.

* Use gender-neutral language. For example, use "chairperson" rather than "chairman."

* Use active voice to put more life into your message by focusing on the action of the doer.

  * Active voice: Tim will cut the grass.

  * Passive voice: The grass will be cut by Tim.

- Active voice: I'd like your research proposal by Friday.

- Passive voice: The receipt of your research proposal by Friday is preferred.

* Use correct grammar, spelling, punctuation, and word usage. These errors lead the reader to question the intelligence or education of the writer. Examples of these errors include run-on sentences, spelling errors, using the wrong word (e.g., affect for effect), and lack of subject-verb agreement (Chaney & Martin, 2007). Some of these errors can be quite humorous, such as referring to a "persona au gratin" instead of a "persona non grata." Although humorous, errors affect credibility. See Table 4.2 for some common writing traps.

* Use humor with caution. Remember that without the non-verbal aspect of the message, the reader may see no humor in what you have written. Your attempts at humor may be perceived as flippant (Chaney & Martin, 2007).

* Use specific and positive statements as much as possible. Rather than saying, "Don't forget to submit your budget soon," say, "Please turn in your budget by Friday, June 13, by 4 p.m.

* Use a variety of sentence types and lengths. The average length of a sentence should be from 13 to 20 words. Limit sentences to 20 to 25 words. As a general rule, use short sentences for emphatic statements and long sentences for detailed explanations. Varying the length adds to the effectiveness of your message (Chaney & Martin, 2007; Lindsell-Roberts, 2004).

* Limit your paragraphs to about 7 or 8 lines of text. When paragraphs are too long, the reader may skip over them. When they are too short and choppy, the reader may not see the connection between ideas (Lindsell-Roberts, 2004).

✳ Use courtesy expressions (please, thank you, etc.) frequently and in the proper place. Some writers end the message with "thank you" or "thank you in advance" when nothing has been done for which the recipient should be thanked. If you requested some action of the reader, express your appreciation in the future tense (Chaney & Martin, 2007). For example, "I would appreciate your returning my map before the holiday weekend."

✳ Replace a dictatorial tone (must or should) with a polite (please) tone. It is so much nicer to say, "Please submit the time schedule" instead of "You should submit the time schedule." Tone—how you sound to the reader—is important in writing. Through your choice of words, you can sound positive, pleasant, or enthusiastic. Comparatively, you can also sound stuffy, hostile, or passive.

✳ Keep it short and simple (KISS). In 1998, President Clinton signed the Plain Language Law. Part of it states that "Shorter is better than longer . . . active is better than passive . . . clarity helps advance understanding" (Lindsell-Roberts, 2004, p.47).

 Examples of Windbag Phrases to Avoid

Windbag Phrases	*Concise Replacements*
Due to the fact that	Because
The reason why	Because
In spite of the fact that	Although
At the earliest possible date	As soon as
Prior to	Before
During the month of June	In June
Conduct an investigation	Investigate
Held a meeting	Met

Windbag Phrases	Concise Replacements
At the present time	Now
Draw your attention to	Show you
After that has been done	Then
There is no doubt	Undoubtedly
Allows the opportunity	Allows
Arrived at the conclusion	Concluded
Until such time as you are able to	Until you can

Communication Coach

A business leader was asked to offer testimony before Congress. He and the White House were embarrassed when it was found that a presidential official had edited his statement. Unfortunately, the business leader did not know how to turn off Track Changes (a feature that shows previous edits). The editing confirmed the existence of governmental support that the businessman and the White House had denied.

Lesson: Word documents may show tracked changes. If you don't want people to see what has been done to the document, make sure the changes are accepted or rejected.

Common Writing Traps

affect and effect

Affect is usually a verb meaning to influence. As a noun, **effect** means result; as a verb, it means to bring to pass.

Example: The new legislation affected mandatory overtime, and this effect helped nurse recruitment.

all ready and already	**All ready** used as an adjective means completely prepared. **Already** is an adverb meaning previously, before, or sooner than expected.
	Example: The new lab reports are all ready to be filed. Some lab reports were already in the chart.
all together and altogether	**All together** means collectively in the same place. **Altogether** is an adverb meaning entirely, completely, on the whole.
	Example: The hospital reviewers were all together in the board room. The conferences were long, but altogether worthwhile.
among and between	**Among** is used when two or more things or people are involved. **Between** is used with only two.
	Example: This matter should be kept between the two of us. This gift should be shared among the entire staff.
assure, ensure, and insure	**Assure** is a verb that means to promise or to make certain by setting a person's mind at rest. **Ensure** is a verb meaning to make secure or make safe. **Insure** is a verb meaning to make secure or to guarantee from risk.
	Example: Maria was assured that she would be promoted by the end of the year. Safety goggles ensure against splashing into the eyes. The cabin is insured against theft or fire.
bring and take	**Bring** indicates motion toward a person. **Take** indicates motion away.
	Example: Please bring this water to Mrs. Miller and take the dinner tray from the room.

can and may	**Can** implies ability. **May** implies permission.
	Example: Jerry may obtain the blood sugar if he can.
complement and compliment	**Complement** refers to something that completes. **Compliment** refers to praise.
	Example: The color of that scarf complements your suit. He gave me a nice compliment about my scarf.
emigrate and immigrate	People **emigrate** or move from a country. People **immigrate** or move into another country.
	Example: The Irish emigrant was given permission to immigrate to the United States.
farther and further	**Farther** refers to a physical distance; **further** means more or additional and is used as a time or quantity word (such as further discussion).
	Example: Please move that desk farther to the right. Let's take the discussion one step further and make a recommendation.
fewer and less	**Fewer** refers to items that you can count. **Less** refers to degree or quantity.
	Example: There are fewer nurses in the same day surgery unit, and they have less experience than the recovery room nurses.
irregardless and regardless	**Irregardless** is not a word and should not be used. **Regardless** means despite or in spite of something.
	Example: The hiring decision has already been made, regardless of what the staff may recommend.

its and it's	**Its** is the possessive form of the pronoun "it." **It's** is the contraction of "it is."
	Example: The hospital has maintained its religious roots. It's time to start planning the induction ceremony.
me	**Me** is the object of a verb or preposition.
	Example: This problem is between you and me. They called you and me.
precede and proceed	**Precede** is a verb that means to come before in rank, or time. **Proceed** is a verb that means to move on or go forward, especially after stopping.
	Example: Mike's voice was louder than the speakers who preceded him. Their family doctor advised them on the best way to proceed after the surgery.
stationary and stationery	**Stationary** means fixed; **stationery** refers to writing materials.
	Example: Once correctly installed, the new mailbox remained stationary. I will write him a thank-you note with my new stationery.
was and were	**Was** is used for things in the past. **Were** expresses a wish or states a doubtful situation.
	Example: I was surprised to find you there. If I were a college student, I would choose nursing as a career.
who and whom	**Who** is used for the person who is the subject of a sentence. **Whom** (the objective case of who), refers to the person who has been the object of an action.
	Example: Who bought the new bed? The new bed is to be used by whom?

(Pagana, 2008)

"The difference between the right word and almost the right word is the difference between lightening and the lightening bug."

–Mark Twain

Business Letters

What is the best way to learn how to write a business letter?

Just as a puzzle is completed by putting all the pieces in the right place, a business letter has a designated place for its components. You need to learn the different parts and where to put them. Listed below are the parts of a letter in the order in which they should appear. Not all components (such as the subject line and enclosure notations) are used in every letter (Lindsell-Roberts, 2004). Letters should be printed on the organization's letterhead.

* Date line: The position of the date depends on the block style being used. (Block styles are discussed later.)

* Inside address: This should be several lines below the date line and include the name, job title, street address or post office box, suite or room number, city, state, and ZIP code.

* Salutation: The salutation should be two lines below the address. The salutation should correspond directly to the first line of the inside address. Formal and informal examples are shown in Table 4.3.

43   Examples of Salutations

Inside Address	Salutation—formal	Salutation—informal
Mr. Dennis Deska	Dear Mr. Deska:	Dear Dennis,
Ms. Leah Fleming	Dear Ms. Fleming:	Dear Leah,
Mr. and Mrs. Joseph Brown	Dear Mr. and Mrs. Brown:	Dear Joe and Alice,
Dr. John Jones and Dr. Veronica Jones (husband and wife)	Dear Doctors Jones:	Dear John and Veronica,
Joel King, Esq. (attorney)	Dear Mr. King:	Dear Joel,
Smith & Carson, Esqs. (one man and one woman)	Dear Mr. Smith and Ms. Carson:	Dear Beryl and Irene,

✳ Subject line: This describes the purpose of the letter. Because it is part of the body, it's placed two lines below the salutation.

✳ Body: The body is the longest part of the letter. Single-space the body of the letter, and double-space between paragraphs. If the body of the message is only a few sentences, double-space.

✳ Complimentary close: Place this several lines below the last line of the body. Only capitalize the first word. Use a comma after the last word. For example:

- Sincerely,

- Sincerely yours,

- Best wishes,

- Kindest regards,

- Respectfully,

＊ Signature line: Place this line under the complimentary closing. Leave enough room to sign your name. Place the writer's
job title on the line below the typed name.

＊ Reference initials: These initials identify the typist if someone
other than the author typed the letter. They are placed on the
left margin, two lines below the signature line. These are not
needed when writers type their own letters.

＊ Enclosure notation: When anything is enclosed in the envelope
besides the letter, place an enclosure notation on the line below the reference initials.

＊ Copy notation: When you send a copy of the letter to another
person, place a notation directly below the enclosure notation
or reference initials. The "cc" is a holdover from the old "carbon copy" although it's often called a "courtesy copy." Many
offices are now using "pc" for "photocopy." If you don't want
the addressee to know that a copy of the let-
ter is being forwarded to another person,
use "bc" for blind copy. This notation
would only appear on the office copy
and third-party copy—not on the
original letter.

TIP

For extra
emphasis, type
the postscript in
a different font
or handwrite
it.

＊ Postscript: Place the P.S. two lines below your last notation. The P.S. initials
can be included or left out.

Communication Coach

In 1802, Victor Hugo sent a letter to his publisher asking how he
liked the manuscript, *Les Miserables*. The publisher replied, "!"
(Lindsell-Roberts, 2004).

Lesson: The less you say, the more you say. Keep it short and
simple (KISS).

Basic parts of a business letter

Susquehannah Health System   <Letterhead>
499 Grampian Boulevard
Williamsport, PA 17701

September 15, 2010 <Date>

<Inside address>
Ms. Ginny Thomas
Director of Personnel
Warminster General Hospital
217 Centennial Road
Warminster, PA 18974

Dear Ms. Thomas: <Salutation>

SUBJECT: Letter of recommendation for Monica Pope <Subject line>

<Body>
I am delighted to write a letter of recommendation for Monica Pope.
She has been employed at Susquehanna Health System as a Diabetic
Nurse Educator for 5 years. We are disappointed that she had to
relocate out of our area. She is well respected here and had a bright
future with us. She played a key role in our achievement of Magnet
Hospital designation.

I am enclosing a copy of a recent award that Monica received during
our Nursing Week. Monica is intelligent, hard-working, and dedicated to her patients. We are sorry to lose her. She will surely be an
asset to your staff.

Sincerely yours, <Complimentary closing>
<Signature line>
Mary Jane Brody, MSN, RN <Writer's typed name>
Vice President of Nursing <Job title>

MJB/je <Reference initials; means that June Evans typed the letter for
Mary Jane Brody>
1 Enc. <Enclosure notation>
cc: Monica Pope <Copy notation>

P.S. Please give Monica my best regards. <Postscript>

What are the most common styles for setting up business letters?

The two most popular styles are the block and the modified block. Semiblock is also used, but not as popular.

* Block style: All lines begin at the left margin. There is no need to indent. The example above uses block style.

* Modified block style: The date, closing, and signature block are slightly to the right of center. Everything else starts at the left margin.

* Semiblock style: This is identical to the modified block, except the first line of each paragraph is indented.

TIP

Don't reinvent the wheel. If you've written letters before for similar purposes, use them for ideas, words, and phrases, and mimic their brevity.

What is recommended for margins?

Letters should be centered with equal left and right margins (1 to 1.5 inches) and equal top and bottom margins. Don't crowd material onto a single page if you have to cut your margins, formatting, and white space.

How important is white space?

White space—the areas of the paper where there is no text or graphics—makes the message easy to read. Here are some ways to create white space:

* Use appropriate margins. Don't cram a lot of information onto a single page.

* Double-space between paragraphs.

* Use lists, charts, and tables when appropriate.

How do you handle the letterhead when typing a multipage letter?

Use letterhead for the first page and matching plain paper for the other pages. Here are two styles to consider for the top of the other pages:

Mary Jane Brody	Page 2	Date

Mary Jane Brody
Page 2
Date

Is there a rule or guideline for dividing paragraphs between pages in a multipage letter?

Yes. When you divide a paragraph, leave at least two lines on the current page and carry over at least two lines on the next page. Don't divide the paragraph if you can't do this. Don't divide a three-line paragraph.

What should you do if your complimentary close is the only thing that was carried over to a second page?

Change the page break so you have at least two lines of text over the complimentary close. You need the text for continuity.

What is the best kind of paper to use for important correspondence?

Appropriate bond is generally 25 percent rag-content and at least 20- or 24-pound weight. White or off-white paper with black ink is preferred.

Do you have any tips for folding and inserting a business letter into an envelope?

Yes. Correct folding and insertion gives the letter a professional look and makes it easy for the reader to open and unfold. Here is the guideline for a No. 10 envelope (4-1/8" by 9-1/2" inches).

* Put the letter face up on a flat surface. Fold up the bottom third of the paper first.

* Fold the top third of the letter down over the bottom third so the edge is 1/4 inch from the first fold.

* Insert the letter into the envelope so it is right side up and readable when removed from the back of the envelope (Pagana, 2008).

TIP

The postal carrier will deliver mail to the address element on the line above the city, state, and ZIP code. If you want the letter delivered to a post office box, place the PO Box number under the street address and above the city, state, and ZIP code line.

Standard State Two-Letter Abbreviations

Alabama	AL	Florida	FL	Maine	ME
Alaska	AK	Georgia	GA	Maryland	MD
Arizona	AZ	Hawaii	HI	Massachu-setts	MA
Arkansas	AR	Idaho	ID		
California	CA	Illinois	IL	Michigan	MI
Colorado	CO	Indiana	IN	Minnesota	MS
Connecticut	CT	Iowa	IA	Mississippi	MS
Delaware	DE	Kansas	KS	Missouri	MO
District of Columbia	DC	Kentucky	KY	Montana	MT
		Louisiana	LA		

Standard State Two-Letter Abbreviations
continued

Nebraska	NE	North Dakota	ND	Tennessee	TN
Nevada	NV	Ohio	OH	Texas	TX
New Hampshire	NH	Oklahoma	OK	Utah	UT
		Oregon	OR	Vermont	VT
New Jersey	NJ	Pennsylvania	PA	Virginia	VA
New Mexico	NM	Rhode Island	RI	Washington	WA
New York	NY	South Carolina	SC	West Virginia	WV
North Carolina	NC			Wisconsin	WI
		South Dakota	SD	Wyoming	WY

Communication Coach

Mark interviewed for a position as an evening supervisor at a large medical center. During the interview he was told that he was one of the final candidates and that if he was still interested in the position, he would need to schedule an interview with the vice president of nursing. When he wrote his thank-you note, he made a mistake and wrote, "I will *not* schedule . . ." instead of writing, "I will *now* schedule . . ." This typo caused an embarrassing miscommunication.

Lesson: You can embarrass yourself and negatively impact your professional image with typos.

Do you have any suggestions to become a better proofreader?

Yes, proofreading is a skill that can be improved by following the guidelines below:

* Check all names, including middle initials, and titles. Is the person's name *Teresa* or *Theresa*? It may not matter to you, but it does to the person.

* Double-check all numbers. It is easy to mistake 14,750 for 14,570.

* Check for misused or misspelled homophones, such as *affect* instead of *effect*.

* Watch for repetitive words. Some word processing systems note this.

* Look for small words that are misspelled. You may type "it" instead of "at" or "is" for "if" and not notice the error. Your spellcheck will not catch these misspellings.

* Verify dates with a calendar. When you type, Monday, October 1, make sure that date is a Monday.

* Check for omissions. Did you forget the ZIP code?

* Check spelling, grammar, and punctuation.

* Print out the letter and read the hard copy. You may detect errors on hard copy that you miss onscreen.

* Read the letter out loud. Rewrite if anything is confusing.

* Read the letter from bottom to top and/or from right to left. This lets you view each word separately and helps you detect errors.

* Scan the letter to check the formatting. Look at the margins, sentence lengths, and size of the paragraphs (Lindsell-Roberts, 2004, Lindsell-Roberts, 2000).

"Brevity is the soul of wit."

–Shakespeare, from Hamlet

Memos

Has e-mail replaced the office memo?

The office memorandum or memo is still being used for inter-office correspondence even though e-mail has replaced many memos. Memos are generally used in a company to transmit ideas, announcements, decisions, or suggestions. They also provide a clear record of decisions made and actions taken.

How does the memo differ from the business letter?

A memo doesn't have an inside address, salutation, complimentary close, or formal signature. Because memos are typically sent to people within the same organization, jargon and technical terms may be used. Also, the tone may be more informal than correspondence leaving the company.

What are the key components of a memo?

Most memos are formatted with the four headings, or guide words, of *Date, To, From,* and *Subject* followed by the body. (See the upcoming sample.)

These items can be in any order. Be specific with the subject line. For example, rather than *Subject: Evaluation,* use *Subject: Brian Keller Performance Evaluation.* The subject line aids in filing and retrieval, too.

The body of the memo is similar to the body of a letter. Double-space between the guide words and triple-space between the subject line and the first paragraph of the memo (Chaney & Martin, 2007). Limit your memo to one message.

Is there a protocol for the To: section?

There are several ways to do this. It is best to follow the protocol of your organization. Here are some suggestions:

* List the recipients of the memo in alphabetical order.

* List recipients in descending order of corporate ranking. For example, the president's name should precede the vice president's name.

* Mix the two systems. List one or two prominent names followed by an alphabetical listing of the remaining names.

* If the target audience is a group, address the memo that way without listing a lot of names (for example, To: All Employees or To: Recruitment Department.)

Where is the memo signed?

There is no designated place for your signature. You can sign your name or initials next to the *From:* line or at the end of the memo.

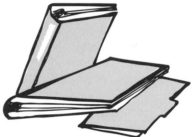

Basic parts of a memo:

(Letterhead)
Date:
To:
From:
Subject:
_____
_____
_____

Business Reports & Proposals

Why are reports an important component of business communication?

Reports provide essential information for daily operations and decision making. Reports must meet the same tests of clarity, unity, and coherence that apply to all good business writing. Correct formatting and presentation are important aspects of report writing.

How are reports categorized?

Usually, reports are classified by length, either short or long. Short reports are called informal reports. Long reports are called formal reports.

What is the usual format for an informal or short report?

These reports usually get to the point in one to three pages and include the following:

* Purpose

* Findings

* Conclusion or Summary

* Recommendation

Some leaders prefer to see the recommendations at the beginning of the report to avoid having to read the entire report.

What are some examples of short reports?

Some common examples include audits, evaluations, incident reports, progress updates, recommendations, and trip reports. Generally, these reports answer the questions of who, what, where, when, and why.

How do long reports differ?

Long or formal reports are more sophisticated in writing style and presentation. They give detailed information and usually require extensive research. They are usually printed on high-quality paper and bound under a separate cover. Often they are externally designed and printed if important enough to warrant the cost.

Formal reports expand on the components of short reports by including some or all of the following elements (Post & Post, 1999):

* Cover page
* Acknowledgement page
* Forward
* Table of contents
* Lists of tables
* Figures
* Illustrations
* Footnotes or endnotes
* Appendix or appendices
* Glossary
* References
* Index

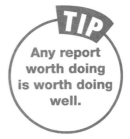

TIP

Any report worth doing is worth doing well.

What are some examples of formal reports?

Some common examples include annual reports, feasibility studies, grant proposals, accreditation self-study reports, product analyses, and research reports.

Thank-you Notes

"Gratitude is the most exquisite form of courtesy."

–Jacques Maritain

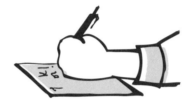

Do thank-you notes have an impact on business success?

Yes, notes to thank someone or acknowledge a gift are an important part of business etiquette. In addition to demonstrating your appreciation for someone or something, you also demonstrate the people skills that are essential for success. Receiving a thank-you note leaves a positive impression that is remembered long after the event or gift.

Is it okay to simply write, "Thank you for your gift"?

No. You should be specific about what you appreciate or the appropriateness of the gift. If a monetary gift was received, acknowledge it with "your generous gift" rather than the specific amount. If you are thanking an interviewer, say something specific about what was discussed or some aspect of the interview process that you especially appreciate, such as being taken to lunch (Pagana, 2008).

What are some other situations that warrant a written thank-you note?

You can never go wrong by writing a thank-you note, but here are some situations that necessitate a note:

* Staying somewhere as a house guest

* Dinner at a supervisor's home

* Acknowledging someone's help with a meeting or project

* Expressing appreciation for an invited speaker at a business event.

"*What comes from the heart goes to the heart.*"

–Samuel Taylor Coleridge

When can a verbal expression of thanks take the place of a written note?

These are appropriate when someone has done a small favor for you. However, anytime someone has spent more than 15 minutes helping you, a written note is in order (Chaney & Martin, 2007).

Is it ever necessary to return a business gift?

Yes. Some organizations do not allow employees to receive gifts. In this case, you would thank them for the gift, explain why you cannot accept the gift, and return it.

Some companies allow gifts to be kept if they can be shared by a group of employees, such as candy or baked goods. However, the employee is not allowed to accept personal gifts.

When should you send a thank-you note?

Sooner, rather than later. Ideally, you should send the note within three days of receiving the gift or attending an event. If you forget to send a thank-you note and remember several months later, send the note. A late note is still better than no note (Pagana, 2008).

Should the thank-you note be typed or handwritten?

There is some flexibility here. If you are thanking someone for a gift or an event, the note should be handwritten unless your writing is illegible. If you are sending a note after an interview, the note could be handwritten or typed, depending on its length. If you want to write several sentences, two typed paragraphs are acceptable.

Some interviewers prefer an e-mail because they get it promptly and can quickly respond to any questions or concerns.

TIP

Don't use a gift or cash the check until after you write the thank-you note.

Examples of thank-you notes:

Dear Melissa,

We had a wonderful time at your dinner party. We loved the food and appreciated the opportunity to meet other members of the staff. Thank you for inviting us and making us feel welcome at Susquehanna Health.

Sincerely,

Denise and Mike Pericci

Dear Ellen,

Our recent Symposium was a great success. Thank you for all of your help over the last 6 months. Your attention to detail and interpersonal skills were instrumental in creating a flawless event. Thanks again.

Sincerely,

Jen McCormick

✔ Checklist

Business Letters

- ❏ Is the message clear and well organized?

- ❏ Is the letter properly formatted?

- ❏ Is the salutation appropriate (formal or informal)?

- ❏ Are the paragraphs limited to 9 lines of text?

- ❏ Are the sentences short, simple, and easy to read?

- ❏ Does the tone reflect my personality? Is it stuffy or conversational?

- ❏ Is the letter focused on the reader, not the writer?

- ❏ Did I check the grammar, spelling, and punctuation?

- ❏ Is there enough white space for visual impact?

- ❏ Are there any coffee or tea stains on the paper?

- ❏ Did I sign the letter?

- ❏ If indicated, did I add an enclosure before sealing the envelope?

Frequently Asked Questions

 Is it okay to thank someone for a gift by sending an e-mail?

Send an e-mail only if you plan to follow the e-mail with a written note. An e-mail does not give the impression that you went out of your way to show your appreciation. It appears to be a hasty attempt to cross something off a to-do list. This is a great example where you should "sweat the small stuff." Most people are delighted to receive a thank-you note. Sending a thank-you note will make you stand out and be remembered.

 When writing the inside address in a business letter, should the person's title appear on the same line as the name or on the following line?

This depends on the length of the line. Try to square the address as much as possible. If the title fits on the same line, use a comma to separate the name from the title. If the title is on the line below, no comma is needed.

 Are there any advantages to using postscripts (P.S.) in a business letter?

Yes, they are one of the first things people read and one thing that people remember. However, if overused, they can appear as afterthoughts or demonstrate poor organization.

If using a subject line in a business letter, why is it placed below the salutation?

The subject line describes the purpose of the letter. It is part of the body of the letter, not the heading.

When is it appropriate to use the addressee's first name in the salutation?

Only use the first name if you know the recipient well and are on a first-name basis. If you have any hesitation or doubts, err on the formal side. You don't want to sabotage your efforts by annoying the recipient with your informal approach.

Is it okay to use "To whom it my concern" as a salutation?

No. This is considered cold and impersonal. Try to find the name of the person you are writing to by calling the company and talking to a receptionist or administrative assistant. You can also check the website.

If you cannot find the recipient's name, can you use "Dear Sir" or "Gentlemen?"

No, sexist language is inappropriate. You could use "Dear Sir or Madam" or "Dear Ladies and Gentlemen." Another option is to address the recipient by title, for example, "Dear Infection Control Nurse" or "Dear Personnel Director."

Does it matter whether the address on a business letter is printed or handwritten?

Yes. Print the address. A handwritten address does not look professional. Printing the address on an envelope can be complicated for many people. It is a good idea to practice with old envelopes until you get it right. Then, put a label on your printer with instructions, such as "Insert envelope front side up and with top toward left side of printer."

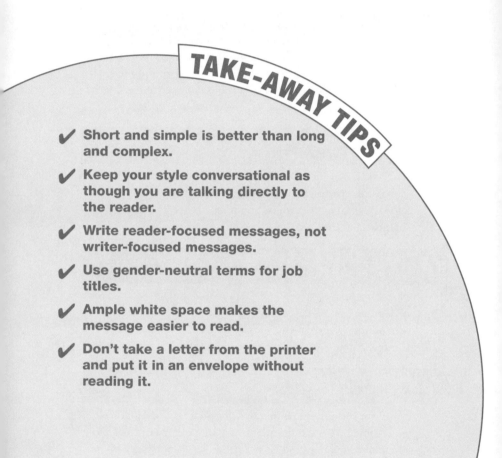

TAKE-AWAY TIPS

✔ **Short and simple is better than long and complex.**

✔ **Keep your style conversational as though you are talking directly to the reader.**

✔ **Write reader-focused messages, not writer-focused messages.**

✔ **Use gender-neutral terms for job titles.**

✔ **Ample white space makes the message easier to read.**

✔ **Don't take a letter from the printer and put it in an envelope without reading it.**

5

✳

E-Mail for Business Correspondence

Do you:

Know what should be included in an electronic signature?

Avoid using e-mail when another form of communication is more appropriate?

Know how to write a useful subject line?

Ever forget to include an attachment?

Wonder how to handle e-mail errors?

Know how to delete your e-mails?

In many business settings, e-mail has almost replaced letters and memos. This raises justifiable concerns about proper usage and etiquette for this popular form of communication. An e-mail message is often the reader's first impression of you. It says as much about you as a handshake. Effective use of e-mail requires additional skills that most of us never learned in school. However, the principles of clear, timely, brief, and precise communication are of vital importance.

"E-mail technology is marching forward too fast for social rules to keep up, leaving correspondents to police themselves and sometimes commit gaffes that would make Miss Manners wince."

--Jeffrey Bair

Benefits and Disadvantages of E-Mail

Why is e-mail so popular?

E-mail is popular because it's immediate and convenient. When used correctly, e-mail has many benefits:

* Messages can be quickly written, edited, and stored.

* Messages can be sent to one person or hundreds with the click of a mouse.

* Informing colleagues across departments, states, or countries is easy.

* E-mail can break the cycle of "telephone tag."

* E-mail eliminates the charges associated with phone calls.

* Recipients can read the messages at their convenience.

* E-mails are cheaper than printing, duplicating, and mailing letters and memos.

* You can write a message any time of the day and send it immediately or at a designated time.

* You can communicate with people around the world.

* You can attach additional information, such as documents, photographs, and spreadsheets.

* E-mail provides a searchable record of your correspondence (Robbins, 2003; Shipley & Schwalbe, 2007).

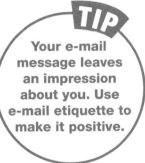

TIP

Your e-mail message leaves an impression about you. Use e-mail etiquette to make it positive.

What are the disadvantages of using e-mail?

E-mail's strengths are also its weaknesses. Being aware of the disadvantages is important so you can decide whether e-mail is the appropriate mode of communication for your message. Here is a list of disadvantages:

* The ease of e-mail contributes to its overuse. This leads to information overload.

* Distinguishing important e-mails from irrelevant messages and junk mail is difficult.

❋ You can reach anyone, and anyone can reach you. This accessibility leads to getting e-mails from people you have never met and also eliminates the once-respectful divide between people at different levels in an organization (Shipley & Schwalbe, 2007).

❋ E-mails lack emotion. Nonverbal cues in a face-to-face conversation or the tone of voice during a phone call convey important information that is missed in an e-mail (Robbins, 2003). E-mails should not be used to convey information (such as layoffs) that requires empathy or support. Conveying emotion or handling a delicate situation is better accomplished with the human voice.

❋ The interruptions of e-mails can eat away at productivity. Opening an e-mail takes time and attention. After being interrupted, getting back to an original task takes time. Some people move on to new tasks after an interruption and neglect the previous task.

❋ Because e-mail provides a searchable record, you can be held accountable for everything you've sent and received.

❋ An e-mail can be forwarded to anybody. Keep in mind that your e-mail can be sent to people for whom it was not intended. Your e-mail message can also be edited or altered without your knowledge.

❋ E-mail formatting can be lost at the recipient's end.

❋ Computer glitches may cause problems with e-mail delivery or receipt.

❋ Recipients need a computer, a modem, and e-mail software. Not everyone is connected.

TIP

If you need to attach a document that you do not want altered, send your message in PDF format or some other hard-to-alter method.

Communication Coach

Dr. Michelle Fine is a highly respected college professor in a nursing department. In and out of the classroom, the students always refer to her as either "Dr. Fine" or "Professor Fine." However, she is surprised when some students send her e-mails beginning with, "Hey, Professor" or "Hey, Michelle." This lack of respect makes her question their professional judgment and etiquette.

Lesson: Don't assume instant familiarity with e-mail.

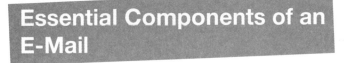

Essential Components of an E-Mail

How can you be sure that your e-mail represents you in a positive manner?

Often we are so focused on what we are saying that we give little thought to the components of an e-mail. Also, many people tend to think of e-mail as casual correspondence and don't give proper attention to the building blocks of an e-mail. Your e-mail can add to others' professional impression of you if you know how to use the following essential components.

* To: Send your e-mail to the right person—the person who can act on it. If you include too many people in your To: field, no one may feel obligated to respond. For example, if you send a message to ten people and ask them to bring a report to a meeting, there's a chance that all ten will bring the report or that only one will. You need to be specific in your request.

  There are several ways to list the order of names in the To: field. You can do it by hierarchy, seniority, familiarity, sensitivity (the person who cares most), relevance to the task, or alphabetical order.

* Cc: People listed in here will get a "courtesy copy" or "carbon copy" of the message you send to the recipient in the To: field. These are people that you want kept in the loop. They probably don't need to respond to the message. For example, if you want to thank one person but you want other people to know about it, you would list them in the Cc: field.

* Bcc: If you don't want the recipient listed in the To: field to know that a copy is being sent to someone else, use the "blind carbon copy" field. Be prudent with your use of Bcc because it's a clear indication that you are sending something behind the recipient's back. If you abuse the Bcc option, this can reflect poorly on you as someone who isn't forthright in dealing with coworkers and peers.

  If you're sending an e-mail to a group of people, put your name in the To: field and list the rest of the names in the Bcc: field. People listed in the Bcc: field get a copy of the message and do not see the names or e-mail addresses of the other people listed there. This protects the privacy of the recipients. You shouldn't share people's e-mail addresses without their permission (Pagana, 2008).

  Be aware that if someone listed in the Bcc: field clicks Reply All, the reply goes to everyone.

* Subject line: This is the most important and, often, the most neglected line. The subject line offers cues for the recipient to know when and how to read your message. Make sure your subject lines say something informative. Always use them and be sure they don't sound like spam. See Table 5.1 for examples of useless and useful subject lines.

5.1 Examples of Useless and Useful Subject Lines

Useless	Useful
Tomorrow	Movie Friday in Muncy?
??????	Tim's vacation visit
Good news	Got a book agent
Quick question	Free for lunch on Friday?
Meeting agenda	Personnel meeting agenda
Urgent	Missing narcotics keys
July 10	July 10 meeting cancelled

* Font: Times New Roman is the font most commonly used in the United States. Arial is the favorite in the United Kingdom. It can be tempting to try to convey tone and individuality by using a more unusual font. Use your common sense and don't let the medium overwhelm the message (Shipley & Schwalbe, 2007).

* Type size: The norm for business is 12-point.

* Color: Black is the easiest to read. When you are replying to someone and want your message to be differentiated from theirs, use blue. Avoid backgrounds or electronic wallpaper for business messages.

* Openings: Don't miss out on using a greeting. "Dear" is always acceptable. "Dear Mary" or "Hi Mary" sounds much better than just "Mary." If you don't know the person, be more formal with "Dear Mr. Smith." Use titles (such as Dr., Professor, Cardinal) as appropriate. If addressing a group, try something like, "Dear Lycoming College graduates," or "Greetings."

* Closings: Because the format of e-mail lets the reader know who the sender is in the From: field, some people don't use

sign-offs. But closings tell each party about the nature of the relationship and tell the recipient how the writer wishes to be addressed. Some closing suggestions include "Best wishes," "Best," "Regards," "Sincerely," and "Cordially." "Sincerely" is the most formal.

Noting how you sign your name provides helpful information. For example, Margaret lets her recipient know her preference when she uses Margaret, Margie, Maggie, or Marge.

✳ Signature block: If you want people to be able to easily contact you, a signature block is helpful. It looks professional and gives people various ways to contact you. See the following table for components of a signature block. Knowing the person's time zone is especially helpful in case you want to connect by phone. See Table 5.2 for components of a signature block.

Setting up an e-mail signature block is easy. For example, if you are using Microsoft Outlook, go to the Tools drop-down menu and select Options. From there, select the Mail Format tab and click Signature. If you don't have Outlook, use your help feature and type "signature."

TIP

Short messages can be put in the subject line. Add EOM (end of message) or your initials after your brief message. For example, "Dinner is at 6. EOM"

If you are writing to someone and do not want the person to have all your contact information, remove your signature block before you click Send.

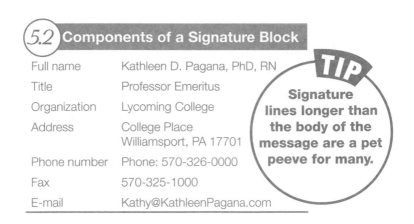

5.2 Components of a Signature Block

Full name	Kathleen D. Pagana, PhD, RN
Title	Professor Emeritus
Organization	Lycoming College
Address	College Place
	Williamsport, PA 17701
Phone number	Phone: 570-326-0000
Fax	570-325-1000
E-mail	Kathy@KathleenPagana.com

TIP

Signature lines longer than the body of the message are a pet peeve for many.

Here is an example of an e-mail signature:

Jane Q. Smith, PhD, RN
Senior Vice President & Chief Clinical Officer
Community Hospital
8796 Healthcare Lane
City, State ZIP
123-456-7890 (work) or 987-654-3210 (home)
http://www.website.com

Communication Coach

Marianne had a long-standing collegial relationship with Tom, the director of human resources at a large hospital. They frequently e-mailed and always used "Best wishes" as a close. When Tom started using "Sincerely yours," Marianne wondered if she had done something wrong and called Tom to schedule a meeting.

Lesson: Your e-mail closing gives a hint about the formal, informal, or changing nature of your relationship with the recipient.

The ABCs of Ccs and Bccs

Cc: I want you to know, and I want others to know that I want you to know.

Bcc: I want you to know, and I don't want others to know that I want you to know (Shipley & Schwalbe, 2007).

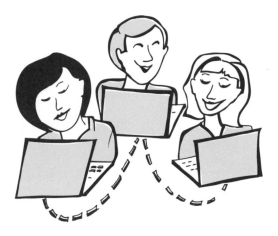

Writing and Responding to E-Mail

"Good manners will open doors that the best education cannot."

–Clarence Thomas

Do you have any guidelines for composing an e-mail message?

Many people have the tendency to prepare e-mail messages on the fly and fire them off to anyone and everyone. E-mail should be treated as an important business communication tool and carefully composed. You should use the same good habits you use for print medium as described in Chapter 4. Here are some points to consider for composing business e-mail:

* Write a short compelling subject line.

* Change the subject line when appropriate as the subject changes.

* Restrict your message to one subject whenever possible. Multiple messages impede the recipient's response and create filing problems.

* Start each message with a salutation.

* End each message with a complimentary close.

* Use a polite and business-like tone. Avoid flaming; that is, sending highly emotional, angry, or insulting messages.

* Try to contain your message to one screen. Think of the questions your reader will have, and answer them in the first paragraph. Answer the who, what, where, when, why, and how on the first screen. If you need a second screen, it can carry the supporting information (Lindsell-Roberts, 2004).

* If your message is longer than two screens, consider sending it as an attachment or posting it on the company's intranet.

* Reply only to those who need a reply. (For example, don't click Reply All when answering an RSVP.)

* Copy only those who need to be copied to avoid information overload.

* Deliver the message in the subject line, if possible. Put EOM (end of message) or your initials at the end of the message so the reader knows that's the full message.

* Use your electronic signature at the end of the message.

* Break the chain for chain letters. There's no place for chain letters in business.

Communication Coach

A graduate student at a southern university had to cancel an appointment with his professor. He sent the following e-mail message: "I will be unable to make our 10:00 a.m. meeting tomorrow morning. Please excuse the incontinence."

Lesson: Proof read carefully. Be careful when spell-check suggests a replacement word.

Are there any guidelines for responding to an e-mail?

People expect a quick response. You should respond within 24 hours. Here are some essential tips for responding:

* Answer at the top of the message. Opening an e-mail and having to scroll to the bottom searching for the reply is bothersome and inconvenient.

* If you are interlacing your response between paragraphs or lines of the original e-mail, make sure your words are easily identifiable (for example, use another font color).

* Make sure your date and time stamps are correct. For example, if your date is wrong, the e-mail may end up in an unexpected place in the recipient's Inbox.

* When a request for information will take more than 24 hours, reply to the message within 24 hours and indicate when you will send the needed information.

* Don't click Reply All unless absolutely necessary.

Communication Coach

An office assistant in the personnel department of an international laboratory and diagnostic company sent a companywide message about an upcoming diversity conference to be held in Germany. Thousands of employees clicked Reply All and asked to be removed from the mailing list for conferences in Europe. This overwhelmed the computer network and shut down service for hours. As a result, Reply All was removed as an e-mail option.

Lesson: Make sure you have a good reason for clicking Reply All.

Should you use the out-of-office feature when you will be away?

Because people expect a quick response, this is a good idea. This bounce back message lets the person know that you are away and unable to respond for a certain time. This courtesy keeps the person from wondering whether you received the message or why you are not responding.

How can you make your message easy to read on-screen?

The informal nature of e-mail makes many people forget the importance of readability. Here are some suggestions:

* Using all capital letters, in addition to being hard to read, denotes SHOUTING.

* Using all lower case letters implies laziness.

* Limit paragraphs to seven or eight lines of text. Space between paragraphs.

* Use bullets and numbers where appropriate.

* Keep messages short. Limit the length to two screens.

* Use normal sentence structure with standard capitalization and proper punctuation.

* To emphasize a word or phrase, place it between asterisks (* . . . *).

Is there a recommended way to forward e-mails?

Forwarding is a great way to pass on legitimate business-related information that may be beneficial to others, but be selective. Listed below are some forwarding tips:

* Forward only what your reader needs to see.

* Decide whether you should change the subject line.

* Eliminate the e-mail headers showing everyone who has received the message and remove the >>>> symbols.

How about using acronyms in business e-mail?

It's okay to use well known acronyms, such as FYI (for your information) and FAQ (frequently asked questions) in business communication. Other acronyms are more commonly used in text messaging and informal communication. Here are some acronyms to limit to informal communication: (Eichhorn, Thomas-Maddox, & Wanzer, 2008; Lindsell-Roberts, 2004):

* IMHO: in my humble opinion

* ISWYM: I see what you mean

* LOL: laughing out loud

* AFAIK: as far as I know

* FWIW: for what it's worth

* PCM: please call me

Is it acceptable to use emoticons in business e-mail?

Emoticons are symbols made up of keyboard key combinations that convey emotion. Don't use them in formal business e-mails. Table 5.3 shows emoticons commonly used for corresponding with your friends. To read or understand emoticons, turn your head counterclockwise.

5.3 Emoticons for Informal Communication

Emoticon	Emotion Conveyed
:-‖	Anger
:-∣	Apathy
X-(	Brain dead
%-∣	Confusion
;-(	Sadness
:)	Smiley face
:(	Frowning face
;)	Winking
:-}	Happiness
:-o	Shocked
:-/	Skeptical
:-D*	Laughing so hard you don't notice a 5-legged spider hanging from your lip

Do you have any guidelines for international e-mail?

Be aware of differences in writing the date in your message. Europeans format the date as date/month/year. People in Japan use a year/month/date format. For example, if you refer to 5/6/10, in the U.S. that would mean May 6th, but in Europe it would mean June 5th. To avoid this problem, write out the month, date, and year (May 6, 2010) because you don't know who may read your message (Lindsell-Roberts, 2000).

Are there any suggestions for handling e-mail errors?

Because of the volume of e-mail, most of us will have to handle errors. Although e-mail can get you into trouble, it typically doesn't get you out of trouble. Here are some helpful tips:

* Pick up the phone and apologize right away.

* Don't blame the mistake on e-mail (for example, spell-check).

* Pray that the other person has made a similar error and is willing to forgive you (Shipley & Schwalbe, 2007).

"Politeness and consideration for others is like investing pennies and getting dollars back."

–Thomas Sowell

Using Attachments

What things should be considered before sending attachments?

The ability to attach materials to e-mail is a blessing and an annoyance. People attach too much and too often. Here are some questions to ask before sending an attachment:

* Is this attachment really necessary?

* Could you put this material in the body of the message instead?

* Can you put this information on a Web page and provide a link?

* Are you filling up someone's server space with large files?

What are some disadvantages of sending attachments?

Here are a few things to think about:

* Attachments use up a lot of server space.

* They can be hard to see on handheld devices.

* They can carry viruses.

* They can be blocked by many e-mail filters.

* It is easy to miss some attachments if the recipient does not scroll down in the attachment box. You can prevent this by noting the number of attachments in the message or subject line.

How important is the name of an attachment?

A useful name adds to the clarity of your message. For example, when I attach a speaker proposal, it is better to name the attachment "Pagana.speakerproposal" instead of "Speakerproposal."

What is the importance of a file extension?

The file extension—the last three or four letters after the period in the file name—refers to the program that created and uses that type of file. See the most common types of attachments and file extensions in Table 5.4.

5.4   Common File Extensions

File Extension	Type of Attachment
.doc	A Microsoft Word file.
.ppt	A Microsoft PowerPoint slide show.
.xls	A Microsoft Excel spreadsheet.
.exe	An executable file. This file will run some program when opened in the Windows operating systems.
.dat	A file containing raw data. This may be unformatted text.
.jpeg, .jpg	An image. This is best for compressing high-resolution images.
.gif	An image format used mainly for photographs.
.bmp, .png	Common image formats for digital photographs.
.tiff, .tif	Tagged Image File that is useful for high-resolution images.
.htm, .html	HyperText Markup Language is used for files designed to be viewed on a Web browser. Most web pages are in this format.
.pdf	Adobe's file format that generally makes the memory allocation of a document smaller. This format is ideal for portability across different platforms.

(Shipley & Schwalbe, 2007)

X *Caution*

People can rename file extensions to sneak them past firewalls. What looks like a harmless PDF could be a harmful .exe file.

Dealing with E-Mail Overload

How can you reduce e-mail overload?

Both the reader and the writer share this responsibility. Here are some ways the *writer* can reduce the overload:

* Ask yourself if e-mail is the most appropriate form of communication. Is a phone call or office visit a better idea?

* Send your message only to those who need to see it.

* Write a compelling subject line.

* Change the subject line when replying or forwarding a message, if appropriate. Change the subject line if you change the theme of the message.

* Don't send personal e-mail messages to business e-mail accounts.

* Delete the unsightly >>>> marks.

* Don't get in the habit of tagging messages as "urgent." If something is truly urgent, consider phoning. People are more likely to listen to phone messages than read e-mail messages.

* Break e-mail chain letters. They contribute dramatically to information overload.

Here are some ways the *reader* can be more efficient with e-mail:

* Check your mailbox at least once a day.

* Don't let messages sit in your Inbox longer than necessary. If you are overloaded with messages, you may not reply to messages in a timely manner. If you want to save a message, move it out of your Inbox and into a folder.

* Delete unwanted messages to free up space for other messages.

* Download files you want to keep. Print only when you need to.

* Routinely scan for viruses. When you download files, your computer is vulnerable (Lindsell- Roberts, 2000).

* Tell your friends not to send personal e-mails to your business e-mail account.

How can you deal with spam effectively?

Unsolicited junk mail is a huge problem that accounts for a large percentage of e-mail. Spam varies from get-rich-quick schemes to pornography. Here are some ideas to try to reduce spam:

* Do not open the message. Even if the message says, "If you'd like to be removed…" ignore it. By responding, spammers will see your e-mail address is live and continue to bother you.

* Contact your e-mail provider.

* Block the sender. (For example, if using Microsoft Outlook, right click the message, click Junk Mail, and then click Add Sender to Blocked List.)

* Consider using more than one e-mail address. Give one to family, friends, and business colleagues. Use another for on-line ordering or public messaging, such as chat rooms.

* Be on the alert for phishing.

What is Phishing?

Phishing (pronounced "fishing") is a type of spam. Scam artists pretend to be legitimate businesses, such as banks, credit card companies, or online retailers. They send an official-looking message saying there is a problem with your account and direct you to a bogus site to resolve the issue. The bogus website looks authentic and asks you to fill out a form that may include your social security number, your credit card number, or some other important piece of personal information. Do NOT provide any information. Contact the business and report the scam.

Privacy Issues and E-Mail

How secure is your e-mail?

Your e-mail is about as private and secure as a postcard. You don't know what system your message is passing through. There is also nothing to stop a system administrator from snooping though your mail (Lindsell-Roberts, 2000).

Do companies have the right to monitor e-mail?

Yes. The Electronic Communication Privacy Act (ECPA) upheld a company's right to monitor its e-mail. This is based on the premise that the company provides and pays for the e-mail; therefore, it owns it.

Don't send any message that you wouldn't want posted on a company bulletin board (Lindsell-Roberts, 2000).

How can you delete e-mails?

This is a complex issue. First, delete the e-mail from your Inbox, and then delete it from your trash. After this, you need to use Sure Delete or another rewriting program to make certain the message isn't somewhere else on a drive but rendered unfindable. If you are on a corporate system with proper back-up, the message is still findable.

"Words, once they are printed, have a life of their own."

–Carol Burnett

E-Mail Alternatives

When is a letter a better form of communication than e-mail?

There is no doubt that a letter or note showing appreciation, making an apology, or expressing condolence is more valuable than the most effusive e-mail. A handwritten note is personal. A letter printed on company stationery is official. Here are some other reasons to use a letter instead of an e-mail:

* When you don't want to interrupt someone. Recipients can pick up and read letters when it is convenient for them.

* When you want to create something meaningful for the recipient, such as a letter of recommendation.

* When you want a document that can be filed or archived.

* When you are handling serious business, such as a registered letter or a subpoena.

* When your material is confidential.

When is a fax preferable to an e-mail?

Although many people thought e-mail would kill the fax machine, this has not happened. Here are several reasons to fax instead of e-mail:

* When you need a true copy of a signature that can be legally binding. The law is in flux over when e-mails can be used for an agreement.

* When you want to send hard documents (such as contracts) quickly. Faxing is quicker than scanning and e-mailing.

* When you want a more secure method for sending a document. However, remember that fax machines are often public and shared with others in an office. Another person can pick up your fax and read it.

When is a phone call better than an e-mail?

The sense of pleasure or intimacy associated with hearing someone's voice on the phone cannot be duplicated with e-mail. Voices convey emotions. Additionally, the interaction is in real time. Here are other reasons to use the phone instead of e-mail:

* When you need to convey or discern emotion. For example, a pause or a strained response to a reference check can hint at a more complicated response than the one being given. You could then probe for more details.

* When you have a short time to contact someone about a change in plans.

* When you need to quickly finalize some details.

* When you want your remote communication to be private.

* When you need to contact someone who has no access to e-mail.

* When you want to engage others and have a stimulating conversation.

* When you want to soften the blow of an upcoming e-mail or letter.

Communication Coach

Jocelyn and Denise were planning to meet for lunch at noon. Jocelyn was annoyed when she had to wait until 12:30 for Denise to show up. When she arrived, Denise said, "Hope you got my e-mail about being late." Jocelyn told her she should have called.

Lesson: A phone call is more appropriate if you will be late for a meeting. How can you be sure someone will check e-mail and receive your message?

✔ Checklist

Business E-Mail

❑ Is e-mail the best medium for this message and this recipient?

❑ Is my subject line specific and compelling?

❑ Is this message being sent only to those who need to see it?

❑ Did I respect the privacy of my recipients by using Bcc?

❑ Is my message visually appealing?

❑ Have I established the proper tone?

❑ Did I include a greeting and a closing?

❑ Did I use spell-check?

❑ Did I proofread?

❑ Did I add my electronic signature?

Frequently Asked Questions

 What should you do if you receive an e-mail message that isn't intended for you?

If you know the intended recipient, forward it. Try not to read any more than you have to. Notify the sender that the message was sent to the wrong address. An incorrect address in the directory may have caused the error.

 If someone has several e-mail addresses, how do you know which one to use?

If it isn't obvious, you can ask or send to all the addresses you have. You usually can't go wrong by replying to the address the message was sent from.

 What do you think about asking people not to read an e-mail you sent by mistake?

It won't work. Most people would be intrigued and read the message anyway.

 Is it advisable to update subject lines?

Yes. This gives the recipient an accurate idea of what to expect. Make sure the subject line matches your message.

 Can you tell if a message comes from a handheld device or a desktop?

Unless someone adds "Sent from my handheld" at the bottom, you usually can't tell. However, if the sender is replying with Microsoft Outlook, the subject line shows "Re" from a handheld and "RE" from a desktop (Shipley & Schwalbe, 2007).

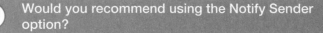 **Would you recommend using the Notify Sender option?**

No. Many people find this annoying. This feature asks the recipient to click a box to confirm receipt of the e-mail. If they acknowledge the e-mail, the clock starts ticking for a response. Many people read the e-mail, but refuse to let the sender know this. This is okay because the box requests notification but does not require it.

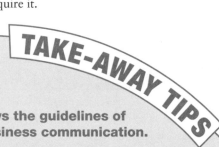

✔ **E-mail follows the guidelines of effective business communication.**

✔ **Pause before you press the Send button.**

✔ **Wait 24 hours before responding to an e-mail that upsets you.**

✔ **Don't expect an immediate response. If you have an urgent matter, use the phone.**

✔ **Never forward anything without permission.**

✔ **Assume everything you send will be forwarded.**

✔ **Keep your subject line short because many people are checking their e-mail on handheld devices that chop off subject lines.**

✔ **Put your e-mail address on your business cards, stationery, fax cover sheets, and everything else that provides your name, address, and phone number.**

6

✳

Writing an Article for Publication

Do you:

Wonder where authors get ideas for articles?

Lack knowledge of the writing and publishing process?

Know how to motivate yourself to begin and complete a writing project?

Wonder how you can develop good writing habits?

Know how to select and target a journal to publish your article?

Know how to proceed if your manuscript is rejected?

Need to develop and improve your writing skills?

Writing an article for publication is something that many nurses would like to do, but few actually pursue. There are a number of reasons for this, but the two most important are a lack of knowledge of the writing and publishing process and a lack of motivation and confidence. This chapter describes the mechanics of the writing process and focuses on motivational strategies to begin and complete a writing project.

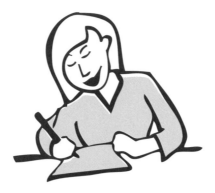

"What is written without effort is in general read without pleasure."

—Samuel Johnson

The Writing and Publishing Process

If you want to write articles, what is the best way to get started?

Approach the process as a learning experience. Nurses are lifelong learners. Remind yourself that you've had to learn many harder things to achieve your position. Accept the challenge in front of you. Tell yourself that you have something of value to contribute that can help others. Take things one step at a time. See Table 6.1 for the important steps.

6.1 The Writing and Publishing Process

Getting an idea

Researching the topic

Selecting the target journal

Writing a query letter, if indicated

Drafting an outline

Writing the first draft

Revising the drafts

Submitting a completed manuscript

Where do you get an idea for an article?

Think of a topic that is of interest to you and would be of interest to other nurses. Don't think you need to be an expert. Your expertise can be greatly enhanced by comprehensive research. Additionally, experience related to the topic is very helpful. If you don't have experience related to the topic, is there something you can do to gain this experience?

If you really want to write, but don't have any ideas for articles, consider the following questions:

* Have you ever wondered why no one has written an article on a certain topic?

* Have you ever searched the literature unsuccessfully to find pertinent information?

* What particular challenges are you facing in your work setting, and can others benefit from your experience?

* Is there a new procedure or technique that you think could be explained better?

* Have you ever written a paper for school and been encouraged to publish it?

* Can you provide a new slant to a familiar topic?

* Can you brainstorm with a colleague to narrow a topic idea?

* Have your read journal editorials to see what topics editors find important?

"Writing comes more easily if you have something to say."

—Sholem Asch

Do you have any ideas for researching the topic?

All professional writing begins with a review of scholarly literature. A great place to start should be the Cumulative Index to Nursing and Allied Health Literature (CINAHL). This comprehensive database for nursing publications indexes more than 1,800 journals dating to 1982. CINAHL is available through most medical center and university libraries (Ruth-Sahd & King, 2006).

Medline is another key source for research. This database was created by the National Library of Medicine and indexes more than 4,800 medical, nursing, and health administration journals free (Ruth-Sahd & King, 2006). Medline was the first online database and indexes articles dating to 1966 (Oermann, 2002).

I find it very beneficial to schedule an appointment with a librarian who can help determine the best subject headings and help broaden or narrow a search. The World Wide Web certainly provides another source for gathering such information as published research, scholarly reports, books, and government recommendations.

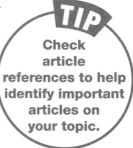

TIP

Check article references to help identify important articles on your topic.

Be open to ideas during your research. Research is stimulating for many reasons beyond collecting data. Research reveals gaps in knowledge, can inspire a new focus for your original idea, and can show you journals in which similar articles have appeared. This can provide you with ideas of journals to target or avoid.

How do you select a journal to target?

Peruse a number of journals. Every journal has a distinctive style directed to a particular audience. The audience may be identified by the name of the journal. For example, the *Journal of Nursing Education* and *Nurse Educator* are geared to nurses in education. Reading through journals gives you an idea of the content and style of a journal. For example, *Nursing Research* focuses on scientific research; whereas *Nursing '10* provides the "how to" about clinical topics.

Use journal survey data to help select a journal for submission and to learn valuable information (journal foci, acceptance rates, editorial style, and reasons for rejection) that can enhance your publishing success (Northam, Trubenbach, & Bentov, 2000; Northam, Yarbrough, Haas, & Duke, 2010). This type of data is published about every 5 or 10 years. See the 2010 reference above for the latest survey data.

After you identify several target journals, rank them from most to least desirable to provide a ranked list for submitting your manuscript. Take into account in this ordering any formatting issues you prefer or wish to avoid. If your paper is rejected, target the next journal (Wink, 2002).

See the following list for the five "rights" of publishing (Plaisance, 2003).

The Five Rights of Publishing

1. Right journal: Did you target the proper audience?

2. Right topic: Is the topic right for the journal? Do you have the knowledge base for this topic?

3. Right information: Is your information accurate? Are your citations correct?

4. Right words: Is your writing concise and clear? Did you mimic the format of the journal?

5. Right time: Is your material timely and up-to-date?

What is a query letter and is it recommended?

A query letter is a letter of inquiry to the journal editor to determine interest in reviewing your manuscript. Some editors, but not all, prefer a query letter. Review the author guidelines found in the journal and (usually) online.

TIP

Generally, a manuscript without a target audience never becomes a published article.

What are the advantages of writing a query letter?

The editor's feedback directs your manuscript toward becoming more publishable. Remember that a positive response to a query letter is no guarantee the journal is accepting your manuscript (Pierce, 2009). The editor can also say your article is unneeded because a similar article has been accepted. Although rejection is disappointing, it saves you time and energy and provides feedback to possibly improve your manuscript.

Communication Coach

Many years ago when I was trying to publish my first article, I followed the author's guidelines and submitted a query letter. I described the manuscript I was writing on jejunostomy tube feedings. The editor responded and suggested that I focus my manuscript on "preventing complications." My subsequent manuscript was accepted for publication after a few minor revisions.

Lesson: Follow the feedback an editor provides in a query letter. This will increase your chance of getting a published article.

How do you write a query letter?

The query letter is a mini sample of how you write. It should be well-written, thoroughly proofread for spelling and grammatical errors, and include the following:

* The correct name and spelling of the current editor

* The tentative title of the manuscript

* A succinct paragraph describing your proposed manuscript

* A description of tables, graphs, or illustrations—if any are included

* An explanation of why you are qualified to write the manuscript

How important is an outline for writing an article?

An outline is essential for providing a visual representation of the writer's thoughts. An outline's detail varies from one writer to another, is not written in stone, and can be altered throughout the writing process (Pagana, 1989). For example, suppose you are writing about a clinical problem and a drug commonly used for treatment is recalled by the Food and Drug Administration. Adding this new information would make your paper more valuable.

Additionally, an outline allows you to focus on appropriate content while adhering to a realistic timeline (Plaisance, 2003). Following an outline provides direction throughout your writing periods. You don't have to wonder what to write next because the decision has been made. Follow your guideline and stay on target.

How can you motivate yourself to write a rough draft?

For many people, the first draft is the hardest and most challenging part of writing. Don't waste time trying to develop great opening lines. Start writing wherever you feel like writing. For example, don't start with the introduction when you are eager to write a different section. Writing the introduction may be easier after completing the first draft of the article.

You don't need to follow your outline from beginning to end. As long as all the sections are completed by the end of the first draft, you're in good shape. The most important thing is to have something written so it can be revised and critiqued.

Do you have any tips for revising your first draft?

TIP

Before writing, review recent issues of the target journal and mimic the format and writing style.

Remember that all good writing requires rewriting. With practice, the writing process can be honed, polished, and refined (Ruth-Sahd & King, 2006). Let a few days pass between rewrites so you have time to be objective about your writing. Consider the following when revising your first draft:

* Did you state what you wanted clearly?

* Is the purpose clear?

* Did you eliminate unnecessary words?

* Is any content missing?

* Is the content logically sequenced?

* Did you design a chart or table to help explain complex information?

* Did you follow the author guidelines?

* Did you follow the journal's format?

* Did you cite and format all references correctly?

* Did you carefully check grammar, punctuation, and spelling?

"Vigorous writing is concise."

–William Strunk, Jr.

What is the best way to get helpful feedback from colleagues?

Don't ask colleagues to critique your work until you've revised it several times. Asking colleagues to read a draft filled with typos and grammar errors is inappropriate. The readers will be too bogged down with errors to provide a good review.

Ask your colleagues to be objective and try to negotiate a deadline for the feedback. Ask them to critique such factors as content accuracy, organization, flow, and level of the intended audience (Pagana, 1989). Often colleagues can suggest an important reference that's been overlooked. Use their feedback to revise the manuscript.

TIP

Revise.
Revise. Revise.
(Hemingway wrote
the ending to *A
Farewell to Arms*
39 times!)

Can you use copyrighted material in an article?

You need written permission to use copyrighted material; therefore, check the author guidelines or contact the editorial staff for copyright questions. If you want to use cartoons, you usually have to pay for them.

What should be included in a cover letter to the editor?

The cover letter should be well written and concise and should describe who you are and why you're qualified to write the manuscript. Most journals require a statement confirming that the manuscript is original and has not been previously submitted or published. Including the author's name, affiliation, and complete contact information is essential for follow-up (Oermann, 2002).

What is the best way to submit a manuscript?

The best way is to precisely follow the journal's rules for submission. Most journals prefer articles be submitted via e-mail or online. Follow the directions and contact the editorial office if you have any questions. Make sure you receive a confirmation for receipt of your material.

How long does it take to get a decision about your manuscript?

Plan to wait about 2 to 6 months. Some journals' author guidelines indicate how long it usually takes to review a manuscript. Resist calling the editor about the status of your manuscript unless an unusually long interval has elapsed (Plaisance, 2003).

Usually, outcomes of the review process include the following:

* The manuscript is accepted as is.

* The manuscript is accepted with minor revisions.

* The manuscript is accepted with major revisions.

* The manuscript is rejected.

What if your article is accepted and you sign a copyright waiver?

This means you waive rights to future printed or electronic versions of your work. For example, your article could be published as a continuing education offering, enabling only the publisher to reap financial benefits (Plaisance, 2003).

If your article is accepted, what is the next step?

Be prepared to wait for an edited version. If the editor has made extensive changes, verify that the content and meaning are still accurate (Wink, 2002). Don't make any additions to the final edited copy unless something is unclear or inaccurate.

Don't take edits or title changes personally. They usually improve your manuscript and make it more appealing to the readership. Be sure to meet all deadlines. Most journals follow a tight publication schedule. Respond promptly to all requests. If you miss a deadline, your work may not be published. If you are having trouble meeting deadlines, contact the editor and try to arrange an extension (Johnstone, 2004).

What are the benefits of publishing an article?

By writing, you share your knowledge and expertise with others. This can make a difference to patients and colleagues (Duff, 2001). One of your greatest rewards is the amount of learning you gain.

Additionally, being published can advance your career with raises, promotions, and higher evaluations. Sometimes authors are asked to give presentations and workshops at conferences.

The personal satisfaction of seeing your name in print is indescribable. Recognition from your peers is stimulating. Because success breeds success, you'll be motivated to keep writing (Pagana, 1989).

What are the most common reasons for manuscript rejections?

Although rejection is painful, consider the following possibilities:

* The journal may have recently published a similar article.

* The journal may have a similar article in the publishing queue.

* The manuscript may not be a suitable fit for the journal's editorial priorities.

* The manuscript may be poorly written and viewed as an early draft needing too many corrections.

* The manuscript may not follow the author guidelines.

* Numerous technical terms and jargon may be unfamiliar to the readers.

* References may be outdated or irrelevant.

* The manuscript may not be interesting to read.

* The writing style may not match the journal's style.

* Content may be considered inaccurate or unimportant.

* The manuscript may read like a school paper.

How do you deal with rejection?

Take a little break after reading the rejection notice so you can view the comments as constructive criticism. Remember that rejection isn't final. Determine another journal to target and revise the manuscript to comply with the style of the new journal. Follow the author guidelines for writing and submission. The process will be easier based on your experience. Know that most authors consider rejection letters as a normal part of the writing process.

Motivational Strategies for Writers

What if you think your ideas may not be worthy of publication?

An important part of writing is developing a positive attitude. Have you ever read an article and said, "I could have written this" or "I could have written this better"? Don't underestimate yourself. Your wealth of information and unique perspective may be beneficial to others.

To advance the profession and advance your personal goals, you must get rid of false modesty. Don't worry. If the manuscript is not ready for publication, the journal editor will not publish it. Learn from the experience and move on.

Is there a way to identify your potential strengths and stumbling blocks as a writer?

I recommend filling out the following assessment form (Pagana, 1989) to enhance your confidence, commitment, and motivation in your writing. You'll discover helpful characteristics about yourself, such as when and where you write most creatively, areas where you may need help, and who may be able to help you.

Writing Assessment Form

My colleagues and I say the following are my areas of expertise:

_____

I'm interested in researching the following topics:

_____

I do my best writing (or thinking) at this time:

_____

I do my best writing in this place:

_____

These people are actual or potential resources to help with writing and publishing:

_____

The following are my major writing strengths:

_____

I need or would like assistance in these areas:

_____

I want to write for the following reasons:

_____

What are some key resources to help new writers?

Reading articles and books and attending education sessions on writing are helpful. However, don't procrastinate and get bogged down with "how to write" books, articles, and seminars. The challenge of writing is not met by reading about it. You must write, write, and rewrite. As for necessary resources, all writers (new and seasoned) need a good dictionary and thesaurus. It is also helpful to follow style guides such as the *Chicago Manual of Style* or *The Publication Manual of the American Psychological Association* (APA). Some of this information is accessible and free online. Other invaluable resources include

* *The Elements of Style* by William Strunk and E. B. White

* *The Careful Writer* by Theodore M. Bernstein

Can you improve your writing by reading journals?

Most definitely. Time spent in this manner uncovers topic ideas and writing techniques. When you read good writing, you become a better writer. Additionally, reading exposes you to different writing styles and helps you develop your style. A lot of what you learn about writing is absorbed by reading and refined by writing and revising.

Can reading good fiction improve your writing skills?

Yes. The more you read, the more likely you'll improve sentence structure and phrasing. You'll also see the value of finding the right word or metaphor in your writing (Schilling, 2005). Unsurprisingly, most successful writers are avid readers (Johnstone, 2004).

Communication Coach

Veronica was well established in her clinical career and determined to write an article. She mentioned her desire to a colleague, Leah, who was an established writer. Leah offered to meet with Veronica and help her. When Leah was asked by a nursing editor to write an article that seemed to fit Veronica's area of expertise, Leah contacted and then supported Veronica in writing her first article.

Lesson: If you want to be a writer, tell others. They may be able to help you—and they hold you more accountable.

How can you develop good writing habits?

Remember that writing is a learning process. Here are some helpful strategies:

* Carry a small notebook or card to write down ideas. You may be working, eating your lunch, or driving a car when you think of a great title, an idea for an introduction, or a great example. Most likely, you'll forget the ideas if you don't write them down.

* When you feel inspired to write, write. For example, you may be researching your topic and come across an article that stimulates you to write your introduction. These spontaneous endeavors are often creative and invaluable.

* Designate a time for writing. Make sure this is the time you feel most creative. For example, mornings are my time. Later in the day, I'm not as creative and I struggle with trying to write. Guard your designated writing time and try to prevent distractions and interruptions.

* Find a place conducive to writing. This may be your dining room or a library. Wherever it is, you need to be productive in that place.

* Plan ahead for your writing sessions. Because starting is often difficult, use the last 10–15 minutes of a writing period to focus on your next session. For example, I try to write the first sentence of the next section before putting my materials away.

* Use your outline. The outline should be flexible and modified regularly while you write. The outline gives you direction. For example, if you become stymied and wonder what to do next, the outline directs you to the next point or section you may feel like writing.

* Proceed incrementally. The process of writing and publishing can be overwhelming. A helpful strategy is to divide the process into small steps. Use a checklist to keep track of your progress. You can use the writing checklist at the end of this chapter or devise something that meets your needs.

* Seek opportunities that lead to writing. For example, volunteer to offer a continuing education seminar. After researching, planning, and presenting, you have the foundation for a manuscript. In this manner, the completed manuscript may be a benefit of providing the education seminar.

* Befriend other nurse authors. Seeing that they are regular people (like you) can be inspiring. They may be willing to mentor you, too.

"Most people won't realize that writing is a craft. You have to take your apprenticeship in it like anything else."

–Katherine Anne Porter

How do you handle frustration during writing?

Try not to expect too much too quickly. Don't deprive yourself of other activities you enjoy. You need some rest and recreation to keep some balance in your life. Plan to take breaks and incorporate some restorative activities (such as swimming, walking, etc.) into your schedule (Wills, 2000). For example, you'll be amazed how much your writing can improve after a short walk.

How do you deal with procrastination when writing?

Recognize you're procrastinating and take steps to stop it. For example, if you are trying to write at home and find yourself doing things unrelated to writing (such as laundry), you may need to work somewhere else. Maybe you would be more productive in a library.

Schedule writing times frequently so you can see that progress is being made. Plan to reward yourself for progress. For example, call a friend or go shopping when you finish a section. Another approach is to have an "accountability colleague" to check in with on a regular basis. You may also plan to send sections of your paper to different colleagues by certain dates (Wills, 2000).

Communication Coach

Mark attended an inspirational seminar at a major medical center about writing and publishing. At the end of the session, while Mark was leaving the room, he told the speaker he was ready to write his first article. Mark then added that he was going to take a grammar course first. The speaker advised him to start writing and worry about grammar when revising the manuscript.

Lesson: If you want to write, start writing. Don't procrastinate.

Co-authorship

What do you think about working with a co-author?

For some people, that is a great option because of the support. Some advantages of having a co-author include dividing the work, sustaining motivation, and being accountable to someone. Disadvantages may be loss of control over the project and difficulty scheduling meetings. However, the advantages can outweigh the disadvantages by having help when you write your first article.

"Nothing is particularly hard if you divide it into several steps."

—Henry Ford

How do you determine the order of names when co-authoring an article?

The first or lead author—the person who contributes most to the manuscript—is listed first. Usually, the lead author is the most experienced writer and coordinates the preparation of the manuscript. With several co-authors, the order should be determined by their contribution to the work. To avoid conflict, this should be determined at the onset of the writing project (Oermann, 2002; Price, 2009) and put in writing.

How can you determine if someone should be listed as a co-author?

Only people who have contributed significantly to the project should be listed as an author. The Uniform Requirements for Manuscripts Submitted to Biomedical Journals specifies that authorship credit should only be given when the author has made substantial contributions to the following:

* Conception and design of the study

* Drafting and revising the manuscript for important content

* Approval of the final version of the manuscript (Oermann, 2002)

Are co-authors responsible only for the section they wrote?

No. All co-authors are responsible for the intellectual content of the entire paper. Therefore, they need to approve the final version.

If you want to recognize someone who helped with the manuscript, should they be listed as a co-author?

No. Co-authors should meet the criteria listed previously. Others who helped are included in the acknowledgements. For example, you would acknowledge people who

* Gave advice on the project

* Analyzed the data

* Provided technical or statistical support

* Critically reviewed the manuscript (Oermann, 2002)

✔ *Checklist*

Writing an Article

- ❑ Did I thoroughly research the topic?
- ❑ Did I read all the references?
- ❑ Did I prepare an outline?
- ❑ Did I determine a target journal?
- ❑ Did I follow the author guidelines?
- ❑ Did I write a query letter (if indicated)?
- ❑ Did I write a rough draft?
- ❑ Did I revise the draft?
- ❑ Did I have a colleague read the draft and provide feedback?
- ❑ Did I revise the manuscript several times?
- ❑ Did I write the references in the proper format?
- ❑ Did I carefully proofread the final draft?
- ❑ Did I follow the journal submission guidelines?
- ❑ Did I receive confirmation that my manuscript was received?

Frequently Asked Questions

What should you do if you are researching your topic and find that it has been extensively covered in the literature?

Include the latest information and research on the topic and try to approach the topic from a different perspective. Consider targeting a different audience.

What is the difference between a manuscript and an article?

A manuscript refers to the original text of an author's work (usually typed) that is submitted to a publisher. An article is a published manuscript. For example, you submit a manuscript to be accepted and published as an article.

Can the query letter be sent to several journals at one time?

Yes. This is an acceptable and common practice.

Can a completed manuscript be sent to several journals at one time?

No. It is unfair for an editor and reviewers to spend time reviewing a manuscript only to have it published elsewhere. Journal editors consider this unethical. Submit your manuscript to one journal at a time. If the manuscript is rejected, revise it, and submit it to another journal.

What options do you have if you do not agree with edits made in your manuscript?

Explain your concerns. Don't accept inaccurate materials. If it is a style issue, the edits will usually improve your submission. If you cannot come to an acceptable compromise, withdraw your manuscript.

 What is a refereed journal?

This is the same as a peer reviewed journal. This means the submitted manuscript is sent out to two or three reviewers who read, comment, and recommend acceptance or rejection of the manuscript. The manuscripts are double-blinded by the editor, which means neither the author or reviewers should be able to identify each other. Peer reviewing improves the content and readability of the paper and the quality and standing of the journal in the professional community (Duff, 2001).

 Are authors paid for writing articles?

Most authors are not paid. However, some journals pay an honorarium for feature articles and continuing education segments. Authors usually receive several complimentary copies of the journal issue containing their article.

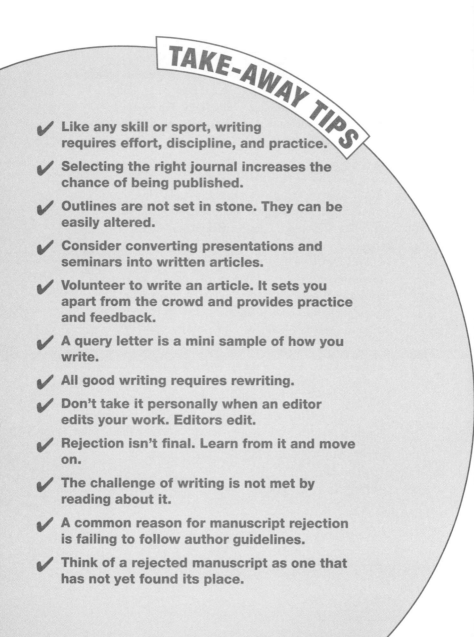

TAKE-AWAY TIPS

✔ **Like any skill or sport, writing requires effort, discipline, and practice.**

✔ **Selecting the right journal increases the chance of being published.**

✔ **Outlines are not set in stone. They can be easily altered.**

✔ **Consider converting presentations and seminars into written articles.**

✔ **Volunteer to write an article. It sets you apart from the crowd and provides practice and feedback.**

✔ **A query letter is a mini sample of how you write.**

✔ **All good writing requires rewriting.**

✔ **Don't take it personally when an editor edits your work. Editors edit.**

✔ **Rejection isn't final. Learn from it and move on.**

✔ **The challenge of writing is not met by reading about it.**

✔ **A common reason for manuscript rejection is failing to follow author guidelines.**

✔ **Think of a rejected manuscript as one that has not yet found its place.**

7

✳

Meetings that Matter

Do you:

Wonder if you should schedule a meeting?

Know the leader and participant responsibilities before, during, and after a meeting?

Consider most meetings a waste of time?

Know how to avoid running an unproductive meeting?

Wonder where you should sit at a meeting?

Respect the time of your meeting attendees?

Routinely evaluate the effectiveness of your meetings?

Meetings are a time-consuming, but vital aspect of most businesses. Meetings provide opportunities to acquire and distribute valuable information, develop team-building skills, strengthen business relationships, and display leadership potential. However, meetings also have the potential to be boring, unproductive time-wasters that result in negative attitudes. These attitudes can be prevented when necessary meetings are well planned and properly conducted.

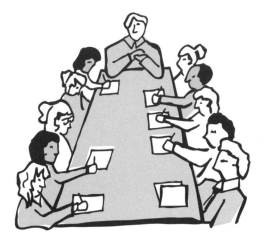

Communication Coach

The faculty in a nursing department was working diligently on a major curriculum revision. Because they were so close to finalizing the details, they agreed to schedule a special summer meeting to finish their work prior to the hustle and bustle of a new semester. They were in for a surprise when the department chair said she had changed the topic of the meeting to a fund raising project and had a guest speaker to explain the project. Needless to say, the chairperson lost a lot of credibility and respect. The faculty was angry with the "bait and switch" during their vacation.

Lesson: Don't change the purpose of a meeting without agreement of the attendees.

"Sometimes I get the feeling that the two biggest problems in America today are making ends meet—and making meetings end."

—Robert Orben

Reasons Not to Have a Meeting

How do you know when not to have a meeting?

Countless meetings are held every day that should not have been called. So, before even thinking about planning a meeting, decide if a meeting is necessary. Here are some reasons not to hold a meeting (Adubato, 2005; Booher, 1994):

* If you can accomplish your goals through a brief conference call or e-mail. Do you really need people physically present at the meeting? Do people need to invest the time and energy to get there and be away from their work for a period of time?

* If you are planning to "rubber stamp" a decision you've already made. If you have no intention of listening to the suggestions and opinions of others, don't bother getting them together. Have the guts to communicate your decision, and be honest in letting them know the decision is not negotiable and their opinions are not wanted.

* If your agenda is not clear. Don't call a meeting unless you have a concrete list of items and issues to address or you risk having a rambling, unfocused, and long meeting.

* If your motive is to communicate a certain message to one team member to avoid a one-on-one discussion. Leaders should not use meetings to camouflage their motives.

* If you just want an audience to hear yourself talk. Committee members will zone out and be likely to avoid future meetings that may be important.

* If you are demonstrating your power to make everyone attend your meeting.

What options do you have if you are asked to attend a meeting that is typically unproductive?

Here are some options to consider that imply you do not want your time wasted:

* Say you are unavailable, and ask whether your attendance at the meeting is important enough to change your schedule.

* Ask whether your attendance is mandatory or optional.

* Ask whether you can send a representative in your place.

* Ask whether you can provide your input by e-mail or by phone (Booher, 1994).

Communication Coach

Every semester the independent studies committee at a college met to review and approve student project proposals. Because of different teaching schedules and office hours, arranging a meeting in a timely manner was often difficult. The new committee chair, challenged to improve this process, sent committee members an e-mail suggesting that they review the proposals and e-mail their recommendations. Members were also asked to indicate whether they felt a need to meet and discuss any of the proposals. The chairperson personally delivered the proposals and a note indicating the deadline for recommendations. Within 2 weeks, all the responses were received and there was no need to meet. So, a process that usually lasted 5 weeks was completed in a timely manner.

Lesson: Explore other options before planning a meeting. Don't be afraid to make a change.

Planning and Preparation

What is the key factor in planning a meeting?

The most important thing is to consider the purpose of the meeting. For example, if the purpose of the meeting is to inform, provide the audience the information and be done with it. However, if the purpose is to generate ideas, get feedback, or make decisions, you need to take a more active role in encouraging participation. Meeting planning (who, what, when, where, why, and how) is more focused when the purpose, goal, or outcome of the meeting is clear.

How do you know how much time to schedule for a meeting?

Timing is critical because you have to consider the purpose along with the time constraints of the participants. Having attendees sit through a meeting for several hours when the purpose could have been accomplished in 30 minutes is irritating. Most routine meetings should not exceed an hour.

"A meeting is an event where minutes are taken and hours wasted."

—James T. Kirk

How is the setting for a meeting determined?

This depends on the degree of formality or informality appropriate for the purpose of the meeting. For example, in a formal setting, the chairperson may select a room with theater-style or classroom-style seating; whereas in an informal setting, the room may be arranged to encourage group interaction.

The meeting site should have comfortable seating, good ventilation, and a temperature level suitable for all participants. People should be able to see any visual aids used and hear what is said. Participants should also not be distracted by something going on outside the room or windows.

TIP

Selecting a meeting room is like choosing a gift box. If it's too small, the gift gets crushed and if it's too big, it rattles around (Lindsell-Roberts, 2000).

The setting should also be accessible and appropriate to attendees with disabilities. For example, chairs may need to be removed for wheelchair access. Persons with hearing difficulties or visual impairments should sit near the front with a clear view of the speaker.

Communication Coach

Ten successful doctors were invited to attend a one-hour meeting at 7 a.m. to share their ideas for improving the health care system. Prior to the meeting, they were given a folder of materials pertaining to the system. The hospital CEO, who called the meeting, arrived at 7:10 and spent the next hour reviewing the material in the folders. Finally, at 8:10, the doctors were given an opportunity to provide input. Because of the time, only two doctors offered any information, and all the doctors left the meeting at 8:30 feeling their time and effort had been wasted.

Lesson: When people are coming to a meeting to help, make sure their ideas are heard and their time is used appropriately.

Chair Responsibilities

How can a chairperson avoid running a bad meeting?

Here are a few common meeting missteps to avoid (Chaney & Martin, 2007):

* Failing to start and end on time

* Showing no enthusiasm and acting bored

* Demonstrating minimal eye contact

* Having a hard-to-hear voice

* Using poor visual aids

* Failing to follow the agenda

* Losing control of the meeting

* Forgetting to schedule breaks

* Recapping information already covered for latecomers

"People who enjoy meetings should not be in charge of anything."

–Thomas Sowell

What are some guidelines for chairing a successful meeting?

Responsibilities of the chairperson include the following:

* Scheduling the meeting well in advance at a date and time that's convenient for most participants.

* Requesting confirmation of attendance.

* Deciding which visuals to use, if any.

* Distributing the agenda a few days ahead of the meeting.

* Starting and ending the meeting on time.

* Following proper parliamentary procedure (such as Robert's Rules of Order) as needed.

✳ Maintaining control of the meeting.

✳ Using effective facilitation skills (see Table 7.1) to create an open and interactive environment so all participants can ask questions and express their views.

✳ Anticipating problems that might bog down the meeting. For example, is a long statistical presentation necessary, or would a summary suffice?

✳ Avoiding recapping information for late arrivals.

✳ Thanking those who contributed to the success of the meeting (those who gave presentations, prepared charts, or arranged for refreshments).

(7.1) Helpful Tips for Facilitating Meetings

Set the tone for the meeting at the beginning of the meeting.

Clearly state the purpose of the meeting.

If a certain person at the meeting has the specific information you need, pose the question directly to him or her instead of presenting a general question to the entire group. This strategy is direct and efficient.

Don't shy away from sensitive but relevant issues.

When people get long-winded or off topic, get the meeting back on track.

Paraphrase and summarize so everyone takes away the same message.

Remember the facilitator is not the focal point of the meeting. The facilitator draws others out.

(Adubato, 2006)

Do you have any tips to keep meetings on track?

Being polite and firm is your responsibility. Try saying something like, "That's a good point and I'd like to discuss that with you after the meeting. Let's get back on track and . . ." Another option is to redirect the flow by asking a question, such as, "Now that we realize the potential problems, what should be our next step?" Stop a filibuster by saying something like, "Mike, I think we understand your concerns. Let's hear from someone else."

How do you handle people who keep interrupting?

You must stop them. Try saying something like, "Can we hold that thought until the Q & A?" or "I think Mark is getting to that point. Can we let him finish?" If the person is interrupting you, say, "Please let me finish." You can also use body language and raise your hand to the interrupter and continue speaking.

Are there any time slots to avoid when scheduling a meeting?

It is advisable to avoid scheduling a meeting early or late in the day, Friday afternoon, Monday morning, religious holidays, or the afternoon before a holiday. People are often busy or distracted at these times.

What should be included in the agenda?

This depends on the type of meeting. An informal meeting agenda may only have a few items for discussion. See Figure 7.1 for a more formal meeting agenda. Formal agendas usually include the following:

* Date and location.

* Start and ending time.

* Topics to be discussed, with the responsible person listed and time allotment.

* If the meeting is scheduled near a mealtime, include whether food or drinks will be available.

WILLIAMSBURG MEDICAL CENTER
BOARD MEETING
Williamsburg Medical Center Boardroom
3–4:30 PM, Wednesday, September 28, 2010
AGENDA

Time	*Presenter*	
3 PM	Chris Schuler, Chair	Welcome & Call to Order
3:02	Brian Williams	**Overview of Board Agenda**
3:05	Mr. Schuler	**Informational**
		Approval of Minutes of August, 27, 2010 **– ACTION ITEM**
		Informational Minutes
		Quality & Safety Committee Minutes, August 3, 2010
		Matters of information / Articles of Interest
		Best in Value Award
		Project 2012 Update
		Pandemic H1N1 Influenza
		Property Acquisition Site Plan
3:10	Margaret Murphy, MD	**Patient Care**
		Quality & Safety
		Satisfaction
		Access
3:30	Margaret Murphy, MD	**Service Partners**
		Physicians
		Recruiting
		Credentialing **– ACTION ITEM**
3:40	Delilah Stroup	**Non-Physicians**
		Recruiting
		Work Climate Survey

3:50	Delilah Stroup	**Innovation & Growth**
		Hospital Signage – **ACTION ITEM**
		Patient Volumes
		Facilities
4:00	Brian Williams	**Financial Parameters**
		August Financial Review
4:20	Claire Wagoner	**Auxiliary Reports**
4:30	Mr. Schuler	**Adjournment**

Figure 7.1 Formal meeting agenda

What is the typical order for items of business on a committee meeting agenda?

The order is usually the call to order, approval of the minutes from the last meeting, reports, old business, new business, announcements, and adjournment.

Why is it important to evaluate a meeting?

This is a great opportunity to learn from mistakes. If you do this while the particulars are still fresh in your mind, you open the door to constant improvement. Determine whether the meeting accomplished your goals. If not, why not? Did you lose control? Did you invite the right people? Did a problem crop up that you should have anticipated? Did you run out of time? Then decide what corrective action you will take the next time.

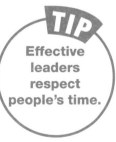

TIP

Effective leaders respect people's time.

Participant Responsibilities

How can you be a productive participant at a meeting?

Come prepared to participate. Avoid any distracting behaviors, such as:

* Doodling; playing with pens or rubber bands; chewing gum; tapping your foot

* Doing anything unrelated to the meeting, such as reading mail, carrying on conversations, checking your BlackBerry, or texting

* Dominating the discussion or interrupting others

* Propping your feet up on an empty chair

What are some guidelines for being a responsible participant at a meeting?

Participant behavior is important to a meeting's success (See Table 7.2). Assume you are there because someone thought you had something to contribute. The following are important guidelines (Chaney & Martin, 2007):

* Respond to the meeting notice concerning your attendance.

* Arrive 3 to 5 minutes early; punctuality is expected.

* Introduce yourself to others and shake hands.

* Bring along your agenda and any other needed materials.

* Come prepared to discuss materials you received prior to the meeting.

* Bring a pen and paper for taking notes.

* Sit up straight and use appropriate eye contact.

* Be aware of negative body language (rolling your eyes, glancing at your watch).

* Give your full attention to the chairperson.

* Listen to and respect the opinions of others.

* Stay for the entire meeting unless you have informed the chairperson before the meeting of your need to leave early.

How can attending meetings be beneficial to my career?

Serving as an effective participant in meetings is an important step in the process of learning to facilitate an effective meeting. It is also a great opportunity to network and to assess information about the organization. If you are asked to volunteer for something, take advantage of the opportunity. How you handle your responsibilities and conduct yourself at meetings can demonstrate your leadership potential.

Is there any harm in arriving too early for a meeting?

Yes, arriving more than 10 minutes before the meeting starts can create an awkward situation for those in charge who are ironing out last minute details or discussing business items. If you arrive early and see that people are busy with last minute preparations, you should step outside and wait until the scheduled meeting time.

What should you do if you know you will be late for a meeting?

Tell the chairperson that you will be late. With advance notice, the chairperson can save a seat for you in a spot less likely to distract others and break the flow of the meeting. When entering late, walk in as unobtrusively as possible and take your seat. Don't rattle papers, get a drink, or greet other members.

What should you do if you need to leave a meeting early?

Notify the chairperson ahead of time and sit near the door so you will be less disruptive when leaving. If you feel that a meeting might run longer than the scheduled time, explain your conflict to the chairperson before the meeting and sit near the door.

 7.2   Leader and Participant Guide to an Effective Meeting

LEADER	PARTICIPANT
Before the Meeting	
Define the purpose	Block time on calendar
Select participants	Confirm attendance
Confirm availability of participants	Define your role in the meeting
Schedule meeting room	Determine what the leader needs from you
Schedule equipment and refreshments	Know the purpose
Prepare agenda	Know when and where to meet
Invite participants	Prepare for the meeting
Distribute agenda	Bring agenda to meeting
Make final check of room	
During the Meeting	
Start promptly	Arrive a few minutes early
Follow the agenda	Listen and participate
Manage the time well	Be open-minded
Limit or control the discussion	Stay on the agenda and subject
Encourage participation	Avoid causing any distractions

Help resolve conflicts	Ask appropriate questions
Clarify action needed	Take notes as needed
Summarize results	
Direct follow-up	

After the Meeting

Restore room and return equipment	Evaluate your contribution to the meeting
Evaluate the meeting	Review meeting minutes
Send out meeting evaluations (if indicated)	Brief others as needed
Distribute minutes	Take action as planned
Take action as planned	Complete assignments by due date
Follow-up on assignments	

(Beebe & Masterson, 2000)

Introductions and Seating

What is the best way to handle introductions?

The meeting chairperson should arrive first and take the initiative to introduce new attendees and welcome regular participants. Another option is to have people introduce themselves at the start of the meeting. If a special guest is present, that person should be introduced at the beginning of the meeting and his or her role should be described. Otherwise, people may be intimidated or distracted trying to figure out why the person is at the meeting. They may be inclined to think the worst (layoffs or cutbacks) unless you explain.

Participants can also demonstrate initiative by arriving early and introducing themselves to others. This provides a great networking opportunity.

How do you know where to sit at a meeting?

If it is your first time at a meeting, it would be polite to ask where you should sit. This can prevent you from stepping on someone's toes by sitting where a higher ranking participant usually sits. Of course, you do not want to sit where the chairperson should sit.

Those invited to make a presentation should wait to be seated until all regular participants have taken their seats. The chairperson will usually indicate where presenters should sit.

Where should the meeting chair sit?

The position of greatest authority is usually the head of a rectangular table that is farthest from the door. This is commonly referred to as the "power perch." This seat commands the most attention and authority (Chaney & Martin, 2007).

The seat to the right of the chairperson is usually reserved for the assistant to the chairperson or for the person next in importance to the chairperson. The person considered next in line of importance usually sits to the left of the chairperson (Chaney & Martin, 2007).

TIP

For a short meeting, try using a room without chairs and conducting the meeting with everyone standing. This minimizes social chitchat, keeps the meeting short, and focuses everyone on the task at hand.

What do you think about using name cards?

Name cards are a great way to learn the names of meeting attendees. The cards should be two-sided so people across the table can read them.

Refreshments

Is it recommended to serve refreshments at a meeting?

Having refreshments is a nice gesture that is appreciated by attendees. Refreshments are usually provided when a meeting is scheduled to exceed 90 minutes. Here are some guidelines to consider when making arrangements for refreshments (Chaney & Martin, 2007):

* Provide a table covering, napkins, small plates, and eating utensils as appropriate.

* Provide glasses or cups for beverages.

* Supply ice in an ice bucket with a scoop for transferring it to glasses.

* Select food appropriate to the time of day (for example, bagels and fruit for a morning meeting; pretzels and cookies for an afternoon meeting.) Avoid anything messy or difficult to eat. It is a great idea to offer some low-fat, healthy food alternatives.

* Offer an assortment of drinks to accommodate various preferences (for example, coffee, tea, soda, and bottled water).

* Confirm your food and beverage order at least 48 hours prior to the meeting. This gives time to correct a miscommunication.

Are there any guidelines for eating refreshments at a meeting?

Remember having refreshments is a gracious gesture. Don't use the refreshments to compensate for a meal that you missed. For example, if you attend a meeting at 3 p.m. and you have missed lunch, don't overdo with the snacks. Make sure everyone gets one snack before you take seconds.

Follow-up Activities

If you are getting short on time during a meeting, should you omit the wrap-up activities?

Omitting the wrap-up activities is like forgetting the closing of a speech. The wrap-up should be considered in the time schedule. The chairperson is responsible to end the meeting properly by summarizing what has been accomplished, clarifying assignments, setting deadlines, and determining the date of the next meeting (if necessary).

What are the responsibilities of the chairperson after the meeting?

The first thing is to ensure that the meeting room is left in good order. Plates, cups, papers, and trash should be removed from the table. The chairperson should then send a reminder to all participants indicating the deadlines for completing assignments. The chairperson should also arrange for preparation and distribution of the minutes. Thank-you notes may be written to speakers, special guests, or anyone who has contributed to the success of the meeting.

What are the essential components of meeting minutes?

The amount of detail and format for writing minutes varies. Follow the format of the committee or organization. Although details may vary, minutes may include any or all of the following:

* Name of group, date, place, and time of the meeting

* List of participants (present, excused, absent)

* Whether minutes from previous meeting were approved (with or without corrections)

* Reports from officers and committees

* Unfinished business and action taken

* Principal accomplishments

* Action taken on motions (name the attendees who introduced and seconded the motion).

* Follow-up assignments

* Date and location of the next meeting

* Time of adjournment

Business Meals

Do you have any suggestions for participating in meetings that include a meal?

Be careful not to let the social nature of a meal overshadow the fact that it is a business event. Your table manners and conversational skills will be scrutinized and will leave a positive or negative impression. You will feel more confident and comfortable displaying proper dining etiquette (Pagana, 2008).

Which meal is usually used for a business meeting?

Lunch is the most popular because it occurs within the workday (not on personal time), is short because people have to get back to work, and is not a concern for inviting significant others (versus an evening meal).

How can you handle the food and still participate in a business meeting in a professional manner?

Be polite and arrive a little early. You may have to get drinks or food from a buffet table before the meeting starts. Avoid eating anything messy. It is impolite to come in late and

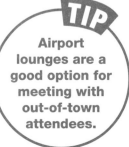

TIP

Airport lounges are a good option for meeting with out-of-town attendees.

distract others while you are getting food. Remember, you are there for a business meeting. Food is not the main priority.

If the meal is at a restaurant, who pays?

The person who scheduled the meeting, regardless of gender, pays the bill and the tip.

Virtual Meetings

Why are virtual meetings gaining in popularity?

Because meetings are costly and technology is providing an alternative to reducing time and money for travel, virtual meetings are viable options for businesses. In addition to minimizing travel costs, they also minimize the human wear and tear that comes with travel. Virtual meetings connect participants by computers, satellites, or telephones. Common examples include web conferences, teleconferences, and video conferences.

What are the advantages of virtual meetings?

In addition to saving time and money for travel, participants are able to share information, discuss options, and often make decisions in the privacy of their offices without being distracted. Other advantages include

* Some types of web conference software generate full text chat transcripts and audio recordings, thus allowing those unable to attend the meeting the option of watching or reading the transcript later.

* Scheduling is easier because participants are more flexible when travel is not a consideration.

* People are less likely to cancel because of personal issues because they can handle their personal business and still participate in the meeting.

* Participants can take turns serving as the presenter without standing up, walking to the front of the room, and plugging their laptops into a projector.

* Large meetings can split up into smaller sessions without needing to find additional conference rooms.

What are some disadvantages of virtual meetings?

The main disadvantage is the absence of nonverbal communication (such as gestures, nods, facial expressions, and other forms of body language). Other disadvantages include

* Decreased opportunities for spontaneity

* Decreased ability for team building

* Compromised confidentiality of information

* Slowing the pace of the meeting while collecting information from participants.

What are the advantages of meetings by telephone or video conference?

They allow real time voice-to-voice or face-to-face communication between people in multiple locations and time zones.

Are there any guidelines for participants of virtual meetings?

Participants need to be thoroughly prepared for the meeting to be successful. Additionally, they need to follow the meeting guidelines, reply to messages promptly, and protect confidential information (Chaney & Martin, 2007).

What things should be taken into consideration when planning virtual meetings?

Here are some important things to consider (Post & Post, 1999; Schindler, 2008):

* Define the purpose of the meeting and invite the right people.

* Timing and notification are critical. Be alert to time zone differences.

* Make sure all participants have been notified and their availability confirmed.

* Send needed materials early and make sure they have been received.

* Provide ground rules, such as when to use the "mute" button.

* Have an agenda and stick to it.

* Start and end the meeting on time.

* Check your equipment in advance.

* Make sure you are comfortable with the equipment or have a support person available.

* Determine a back-up plan in case of equipment failure. (Will you postpone the meeting? Will you use back-up technology?)

* If you are participating in a video conference, pay attention to how you dress and your body language.

TIP

Place photos and short biographies of meeting participants online or distribute the information with the minutes.

What factors should be considered when participants live in different time zones?

It is important to meet during people's normal working hours. The organizer should be aware of how the meeting time affects the attendees' schedules, such as encroaching into their lunch times, requiring they arrive at work extra early, or keeping them at work late (Schindler, 2008).

What are examples of common ground rules for virtual meetings?

Here are some ideas to consider (Schindler, 2008):

* Log on at a specified time (often 10–15 minutes) before the meeting because some online products require downloads and installation.

* Be aware of and minimize background noise.

* Before saying anything, identify yourself every time.

* Participate fully, and avoid multitasking.

* Turn off cell phones and PDAs.

Are there any benefits to not using the "mute" button during a meeting?

Some meetings are more spontaneous and productive if people can readily participate verbally without a pause. Not using the "mute" button also can give facilitators a better sense of whether participants are alert and engaged.

Is it okay to put your phone on hold during a teleconference?

Be careful about doing this. If using a company phone, people may hear your company's infomercial while on hold (Schindler, 2008).

Do you have any guidelines for selecting technology for virtual meetings?

Select the type that best supports the goals of your meeting (problem solving, team building, generating ideas, etc.). Make sure your technology supports your meeting instead of driving it.

✔ *Checklist*

Meeting Evaluation

❑ The purpose of the meeting was clearly defined.

❑ The agenda was prepared and distributed prior to the meeting.

❑ Only the appropriate and necessary people were invited to the meeting.

❑ The meeting room was comfortable and adequate for the number of participants.

❑ The meeting began on time and had a scheduled ending time.

❑ Time was used wisely during the meeting.

❑ All participants had a chance to provide ideas and views.

❑ Participants listened attentively to each other.

❑ No one dominated the discussion.

❑ The meeting ended on time.

❑ If used, audiovisual equipment was in good working order.

❑ Minutes were provided to all participants following the meeting.

❑ The leader followed up with participants on action agreed to during the meeting.

Frequently Asked Questions

 If your meeting is going well and you are out of time, is it wise to continue?

No, don't assume you have the general consensus to continue. Often, people react to ending times as psychological breaking points. When the clock ticks over the allotted time, their minds begin to wander, they lose attention, and they may start to feel resentful. Only continue a meeting if it is agreeable to all attendees. Otherwise, determine the best time to reconvene (Post & Post, 1999).

 If you are meeting to resolve a conflict, do you have any suggestions for location?

Aim for a neutral spot that doesn't favor any of the participants.

 If you attend regular meetings, is it best to sit in the same seat?

No. For the purpose of team building, don't always sit near the same people. This also prevents the formation of cliques.

Do you have any suggestions for keeping people on track at meetings?

This is a critical role of the meeting leader. Some people respond to body language, such as eye contact and gestures. Others need a more direct approach. For example, if one person is dominating the conversation, try saying, "Why don't we hear from someone else?" or "It's time to move on."

How often do you need to schedule breaks during a meeting?

No one should be expected to sit longer than 90 minutes. Provide breaks so people can stretch their legs and clear their heads.

 If you are giving a break, what is the best way to get people back?

Rather than announcing a 10-minute break, tell participants the exact time the meeting will resume. Use the clock in the room. In the absence of a clock, tell people the time on your watch so they can adjust accordingly.

 What is a resolution, and why are they used?

A resolution is a formal statement of the group, approved by a group vote. Resolutions are usually used for achievements, sympathy, or special events. Each paragraph begins with *WHEREAS* or *RESOLVED*, either in capital letters or underlined.

 How do you deal with people who tend to pop in and out of the meeting room?

Close the door after putting up a sign saying, "Meeting in progress. Do not disturb."

TAKE-AWAY TIPS

✔ If people know you start meetings on time, they are more likely to be on time.

✔ Before calling a meeting, determine whether the meeting is really necessary.

✔ Meetings should last long enough to accomplish business—and not a moment longer.

✔ Without an agenda, a meeting lacks order and may not accomplish its purpose.

✔ Bring extra copies of the agenda to the meeting in case attendees forget theirs.

✔ Remember the three "Ps" for attending a meeting: preparation, punctuality, and participation (Brody, 2005).

✔ It's okay to finish a meeting earlier, but not later.

✔ If taking minutes, transcribe them as soon as possible after the meeting.

8

Inter- and Intra-Generational Communication

By Cindy Saver

Do you:

Know the communication patterns of different generations?

Understand how different work values affect the workplace?

Know how to leverage differences in communication?

Know how to best communicate with each generation?

Understand how motivation varies among generations?

The differences among four generations (Veterans, Baby Boomers, Generation X, and Generation Y) of nurses working side-by-side in today's workplace create both challenges and opportunities. For example, a nurse of a generation that values a strong work ethic may resent a younger-generation nurse's refusal to work overtime because it's not in line with the value of work/life balance. On the other hand, a nurse of a younger generation can benefit from the wisdom of a nurse of a generation that values teaching.

Whatever generation you call home, at work you have to bridge the generation gaps to effectively communicate with others. Otherwise, unresolved conflicts could lead to errors, unproductive time, and reduced staff and patient satisfaction (Kramer, 2010).

This chapter explains the work values of different generations to help you better communicate and promote a more satisfying workplace. Descriptions of generations are generalizations and guides, not hard-and-fast rules. Use this information as a start, but don't stereotype. You may be surprised to find that some Baby Boomers are far more proficient at Twitter than their younger counterparts!

"That which becomes the height of absurdity in one generation often becomes the height of wisdom in the next."

–John Stuart Mill

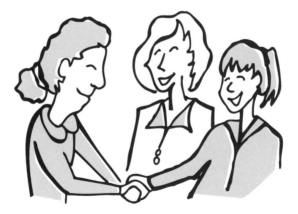

Generations in the Workplace

What is a generation?

A generation is a cohort of people born within 20 years. They share common events, culture, and parental approaches during their childhood and teen years that contribute to their values and outlook on life. Howe and Strauss are associated with the in-depth analysis of generations, beginning with their first book, *Generations* (1992). They state that society is cyclical and that the generations within each cycle have different personalities.

Weren't there always different generations in the workplace? Why talk about it now?

For the first time in history, four generations are together in the workplace (Coates, 2006), from those in their 20s to their 80s, a spread of more than 60 years. Conflicting work values and communication patterns of generations have created challenges. For example, some older bosses feel their younger workers aren't loyal to the organization and need constant positive reinforcement. Conversely, some younger workers believe those bosses are rigid and set in their ways. There is a lack of understanding all around that can be corrected by knowing the sources of differences.

What are the four generations?

The four generations are Veterans, Baby Boomers, Generation X, and Generation Y. See Table 8.1 for some differences among them.

8.1 Generations

Generation/Birth Years	Key Events	Cultural Influences	Parental Influences
Veterans (also called the Silent Generation and Traditionalists) 1925–1945 (38.6 million)	Great Depression World War II Korean War Cuban missile crisis First man in space	Rise of labor unions Golden Age of radio and movies Era of national pride	Reared by authoritarian, overprotective parents who expected obedience and "proper behavior"
Baby Boomers 1946–1964 (78.3 million)	Vietnam War Space Race Assassinations of John F. Kennedy, Robert Kennedy, and Martin Luther King, Jr. Woodstock Watergate	Civil Rights Movement Women's Liberation Movement Television Rock and roll Drug use "Hippies" and flower children	Were doted on by their parents; tend to think of themselves as special and the "stars of the show;" typically reared by two parents

Generations

Generation/Birth Years	Key Events	Cultural Influences	Parental Influences
Generation X 1965–1979 (62 million)	Explosion of the space shuttle Challenger	More savvy about alternative life styles; ethnically diverse friends	Most grew up with both parents working, but also saw adult layoffs because of reengineering and corporate restructuring
	AIDS epidemic	More single-parent households	
	Fall of the Berlin Wall	MTV debuts	Came home from school to empty houses (hence the term "latchkey generation"); cooked snacks in microwave ovens; entertained themselves with video games
	Greater participation in the workforce by women	Technological developments (e.g., video games, cordless phones, Internet)	
	Oklahoma City bombing	Exposure to television violence and adult subjects before they could fully understand them	Resulted in high level of self-reliance

Generations

Generation/Birth Years	Key Events	Cultural Influences	Parental Influences
Generation Y (also called Generation Next, Net Generation, or Millennials) 1980–2001 (92 million)	Columbine High School and other school shootings September 11 terrorist attack (and other terrorist attacks in the world) Iraq and Afghanistan wars Enron and other corporate scandals	Widespread Internet connectivity and community Random violence Globalization and acceptance of diversity Environmental concerns Body piercings	Grew up with lots of praise from parents (and teachers) for every behavior Working parents had more support than other generations; could spend more time with children Respect and admiration for parents; close family relationships are key to happiness

(Alsop, 2008; Winograd & Hais, 2008; Siela, 2006; Erickson 2008; Coates, 2006; Lower, 2007; Weston, 2006)

What is the average age of each generation?

The average age in 2008 was

* Veterans: 63+

* Baby Boomers: 44–62

* Gen X: 28–42

* Gen Y: 12–27

(Erickson, 2008)

It seems like there are a lot of people from Gen Y in the world. Is it just a perception?

No. Gen Y is the largest employee group in history, and equals Baby Boomers in the general workforce (Erickson, 2008). Gen Y is about three times the size of Gen X (Coates, 2006), and there are slightly less than 1 billion more Gen Yers than Baby Boomers (Erickson, 2008). Gen Y is the largest generational group in history, making them highly influential (Erickson, 2008).

What percentages of generations make up the workforce?

According to analysis from the research firm RainmakerThinking (2007) the general workforce is

* 7% Veterans (declining)

* 42% Baby Boomers

* 30% Gen X

* 23% Gen Y (fastest growing segment)

"Each new generation born is in effect an invasion of civilization by little barbarians, who must be civilized before it is too late."

–Thomas Sowell

Generational Work Differences

How do the generations differ in the workplace?

Each generation brings a unique perspective to work. See Table 8.2 for a comparison. Again, these are general characteristics, and some are evolving. Gen Y's desire for jobs with more responsibility has been growing since 1997 and is now at 66% for young women and 67% for young men (Galinsky, Aumann, & Bond, 2009).

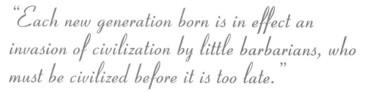

8.2	Generations at Work
Generation	**Work Characteristics**
Veterans	Loyal
	Hard working
	Dependable
	Respect authority and "chain of command"
	Value stability and applying rules uniformly
	Value money as a sign of achievement
Baby Boomers	Skeptical of authority
	Resist hierarchy to some extent
	Idealistic
	Competitive, driven
	Like to teach and learn
	Like team work

Gen X	Value self-reliance
	Need to be recruited each day
	Entrepreneurial
	Rely more on friends than institutions
	Irreverent humor
	May resent Gen Y
	Less collaborative, more pessimistic
	Good "out of the box" thinkers
Gen Y	Like to "figure things out" themselves
	Like the idea of being with one or two companies
	Confident, optimistic
	Want challenge but not responsibility
	Interesting, meaningful work is important
	Like group/team work, win-win
	Not used to planning ahead
	Can multitask
	Like safety, security, and feedback
	Don't want to pay dues
	Don't like hierarchy, not in awe of authority

(Alsop, 2008; Winograd & Hais, 2008; Siela, 2006; Erickson 2008; Coates, 2006; Lower, 2007; Weston, 2006)

A common complaint of nurses from the Veteran generation is that younger nurses won't pull their share of extra shifts. Why is that?

Veterans and Baby Boomers have a strong work ethic, are highly dedicated, and are willing to accept extra hours. Conversely, younger generations value a balance between work and personal life and have no problems declining an extra shift (Sudeheimer, 2009). In fact, Gen

Xers believe that if managers were committed to their staff, they would find a solution to the staffing issue.

Why are Gen Yers less eager to focus on advancing in their careers?

Gen Yers may live beyond 120 years and have a long career (Erickson, 2008). They feel they have time to explore and "try things out." Perhaps this is one reason why they don't focus on moving up the ladder. It may also be why almost half say they would not work for an organization that doesn't offer myriad career paths (Erickson, 2008).

Why does Gen X seem more pessimistic about organizations?

Gen Xers who grew up watching their parents being laid off believe loyalty doesn't matter. Tamara Erickson, author of *Plugged in: The Generation Y Guide to Thriving at Work* and a *Harvard Business Review* blogger (2008), notes that Gen Xers often have conservative work styles and are resistant at work, creating roadblocks.

Why do Gen Xers seem to resent Gen Yers?

Gen X waited behind Baby Boomers for their turn at work. Now Gen Y is coming in much greater numbers and with more technology skills (Erickson, 2008). Erickson (2008) points out that Gen X is the "sandwich generation" between Baby Boomers and Gen Y.

Why does Gen Y need so much feedback?

Gen Yers grew up with an incredible amount of attention paid to them. They received blue ribbons for participating, not winning, and have been told repeatedly how special they are. They have hundreds or even thousands of friends from whom they receive regular feedback (Erickson, 2008). When Gen X was coming of age in the

1970s, fewer than 500 books on self-esteem were published. Compare that to more than 9,000 published during the 1980s and 1990s when Gen Yers were coming of age (Twenge, 2006).

Communication Coach

Andrea, of Gen Y, was enjoying her new job as a nurse on a medical unit. She liked the level of technology and having fun with her coworkers. After 5 days, however, her Veteran preceptor, Pat, noticed that Andrea seemed withdrawn and not as outgoing as she had been. When Pat asked Andrea whether there was a problem, she learned that Andrea didn't believe that Pat thought she was doing a good job. Pat had met with Andrea every day to provide feedback, but discovered that Andrea expected frequent feedback throughout the day. After Pat started communicating multiple times, Andrea returned to her enthusiastic self.

Lesson: Give frequent feedback to Gen Yers (Alsop, 2008). As Marc Prensky (2001) wrote of *digital natives*—those born in 1990 or later (putting them in Gen Y)—"They thrive on instant gratification and frequent rewards."

How do different generations in the workplace perceive each other?

See Table 8.3 for different perspectives by generation. For each generation in the first column, read how it perceives the other generations (Sherman, personal communication, 2010).

8.3		Generational Perspectives		
	Veterans	*Baby Boomers*	*Gen X*	*Gen Y*
Veterans		Self-absorbed	Don't value education, experience, and hard work	Don't take their job seriously; will grow out of it
Baby Boomers	Dictatorial; rigid		Slackers; don't wait their turn	Too dependent on parents, don't play by the rules; both admire and resent them
Gen X	Too set in their ways; they, too, shall pass	Workaholics; need to lighten up		Too positive; need to pay their dues; here just when the good jobs are opening up; are outnumbered by them.
Gen Y	Good leaders, but rigid	Cool and experienced, but work too much; positive view because associated with their parents	Depressed; not sympathetic to their views; not as experienced as Baby Boomers	

Communication Coach

Baby Boomer Lori looked forward to working with Gen Y Anne on her project to incorporate a new laser into the operating room. While dividing the responsibilities, Lori encouraged Anne to take on the technical aspects of the project—learning how to operate and troubleshoot the laser. Lori overheard another nurse saying how Anne didn't like working with Lori. When Lori spoke with Anne, she learned Anne wasn't comfortable working with technology and wanted to focus more on the implementation schedule.

Lesson: Don't assume that the general characteristics of each generation represent each person.

"The old believe everything; the middle-aged suspect everything; and the young know everything."

—Oscar Wilde

Building on Commonalities among Generations

How can people work with others who have such different values?

Focus on similarities instead of differences. For example, we all share 99.99 % of our genes (Bolte Taylor, 2007). Think about it. Only a very small percentage of our genetic makeup accounts for all our diversity. Are we really that different?

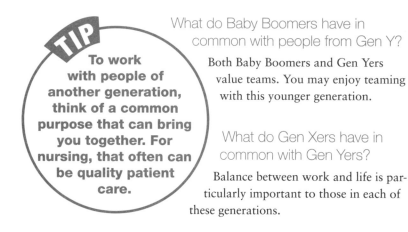

To work with people of another generation, think of a common purpose that can bring you together. For nursing, that often can be quality patient care.

What do Baby Boomers have in common with people from Gen Y?

Both Baby Boomers and Gen Yers value teams. You may enjoy teaming with this younger generation.

What do Gen Xers have in common with Gen Yers?

Balance between work and life is particularly important to those in each of these generations.

What does each generation really want at work?

Surprisingly, everyone wants the same thing, which can be summed up by the 3 Rs and 3 Cs (Stanton Smith, 2008).

3 Rs: Everyone wants to be

1. Respected: To have interesting, meaningful, enjoyable work; to have some control over one's life; to be trusted and able to trust one's leaders; to be loyal and have that loyalty returned

2. Recognized: To be recognized both monetarily and nonmonetarily for accomplishments

3. Remembered: To be remembered as having made a difference

3 Cs: Everyone wants to be

1. Coached: To be coached instead of focusing on finding fault

2. Consulted: To be consulted on things that will affect them

3. Connected: To be connected to their employer and its mission

These seem basic and achievable. The challenge is that generations differ in how they achieve them.

What work incentives are important to nurses of different generations?

According to a study by the Nurse Incentives Project (Wieck, Dols, & Northam, 2009), incentive scores, which reflect the summary of benefits the nurse wants and considers important, among generations were similar. However, they differed in disincentive scores, which reflect the summary of items the nurses thought were important but didn't have. At the top of the list of incentives was a cohesive environment where coworkers pull together as a team—sharing the work and helping each other. Gen Xers and Gen Yers ranked overtime and premium pay among their most important incentives while the Boomers and Veteran nurses stressed pension and retirement benefits (Wieck, Dols, & Northam, 2009).

Many Gen Yers question the need for writing skills when so much is shared in short communications. Do you agree?

No. They still need to communicate their ideas clearly in writing to others. Writing skills boost thinking skills, help people better understand others' points of views, and help people present their opinions in a persuasive way. It has been noted that many Gen Y students cannot interpret information accurately or develop persuasive arguments (Erickson, 2008).

Communication Styles

How do different generations like to receive information?

Veterans prefer face-to-face interactions. Baby Boomers prefer face-to-face or telephone, but find e-mail acceptable. The younger generations prefer electronic communications. One study found that Gen Yers prefer mobile texting, with half using their personal mobile device for texting at work (Information Outlook, 2009). E-mail remains the most common collaboration tool at work. If you send a document by e-mail to a Gen Yer, don't expect a response (Erickson, 2008).

TIP

Whenever possible, communicate in a variety of ways, including e-mail, bulletin boards, blogs, Twitter, and face-to-face. That way, you will be meeting everyone's preferred style.

What is the best way to communicate with Gen Yers?

Keep in mind how Gen Yers use technology. According to Erickson (2008), they send text messages to coordinate or address immediate needs, share general information and photos on a social media site (such as Facebook), and leave phone messages only for someone's parent.

Communication Coach

After 25-year-old Jane interviewed for her first job out of nursing school, the recruiter shook her hand and thanked her for coming. When the recruiter later offered Jane the job, she was appalled to learn that Jane wanted to first discuss the matter with her parents. The recruiter was unsure if she wanted Jane to work for the hospital after all.

Lesson: This experience is not unusual. Gen Yers are very close to their parents. Half of those outside the home see parents daily and 80% talked with parents in the past day (Erickson, 2008). The lesson is to understand the Gen Yers perspective of parental consult is normal for that generation. However, Gen Yers should usually refrain from mentioning their parents in interviews.

How should nurse educators tailor their teaching strategies for different generations?

Use varying techniques to meet each generation's preferred style of learning. For example, you may supplement a class, which appeals to Veterans and Baby Boomers, with an experiential lab session that appeals to Gen X and Gen Y. Here is a summary of learning styles by generation:

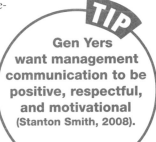

Gen Yers want management communication to be positive, respectful, and motivational (Stanton Smith, 2008).

* Veterans like structured teaching. Invite questions from them.

* Baby Boomers like more formal group learning, less self-study, and teamwork during training sessions.

* Gen Xers want to focus on what they need to know and enjoy experiential learning.

* Gen Yers like experiential learning and multimedia. Similar to Baby Boomers, they enjoy learning in groups. Gen Yers require plenty of feedback. They tend not to think linearly so keeping pace with them can be a challenge.

What teaching strategies are helpful for each generation?

Several strategies can be matched to each generation (HCPro, Inc., 2009; Coates, 2006):

* Veterans: Provide handouts of key points, explain how new skills relate to job performance, and encourage discussion

* Baby Boomers: Incorporate team-building activities and discussions in learning, keep role playing to a minimum, and make information easily accessible

* Gen X: make learning fun, use role playing, allow time for discussion, and use visual illustrations instead of printed material

* Gen Y: give them opportunities to interact, incorporate fun and games, establish a mentor program, provide written resources, provide distance-learning opportunities, and be visual (Gen Y is the most visual of all the generations.)

How does technology affect how Gen Yers learn?

Marc Pensky (2001) used "digital natives" to describe those who grew up with technology as opposed to "digital immigrants" who learned technology later in life. According to the Pew Internet & American Life Project (Rainie, 2009), digital natives were born in 1990 or later, which places them in Gen Y. Digital natives thrive on using technology, which means teachers need to determine how to incorporate technology into teaching.

TIP

Don't ask Veterans or Baby Boomers to demonstrate an unfamiliar skill. They do not like showing a lack of knowledge in public.

One technique Pensky recommends is creating games. For example, having students role-play the Wannsee Conference—the meeting of Nazi leaders to discuss policies related to the Jews—to learn about the Holocaust. Nursing schools are starting to take this on by opening simulation labs where students can role-play a clinical experience.

Do generations process information differently?

Yes. Veterans and Baby Boomers tend to be linear learners, so will read manuals or attend class to obtain information before starting a project (Erickson, 2008). Gen Yers are "on-demand" learners who figure out things as they go. Gen Yers use personal contacts with relevant expertise and may be bored with a long training phase. Gen Xers and Baby Boomers may be annoyed at Gen Yers' frequent questions, but this is one way they process information.

How do digital natives think differently?

Pensky (2001) writes that the thinking patterns of digital natives differ from digital immigrants. They can learn, for example, while watching TV or listening to music because they have honed that skill over the years. They are used to instantaneously accessing the information they need, whether by texting, downloading, or accessing the Web (Pensky, 2001). Other generations need to understand that digital natives won't patiently listen to a discourse on what other generations feel is important. Their roving minds need to be kept active. They prefer multitasking.

So, technology is the problem, right?

Not really. Technology itself isn't the problem. The problem is how different generations interpret each other's communication intentions (Erickson, 2009). Generation X and Y expect a quick response from their peers, so they may feel frustrated or rejected if they don't hear from their older colleagues for a day. Veterans may feel left out when there is no face-to-face communication (Erickson, 2009). Balance in communication styles is the key.

"Education is simply the soul of a society as it passes from one generation to another."

–G.K. Chesterton

Leveraging Differences

How can nurse managers build project teams that communicate and work effectively?

One strategy is to leverage the differences among the generations by mixing the team. Consider what each generation brings to the table (Hobbs, 2005):

* Veterans bring wisdom based on their years of experience and an understanding of the historical background of an issue.

* Baby Boomers bring their clinical and organizational experience.

* Gen Xers bring innovative ideas and creative approaches.

* Gen Yers bring technological expertise.

Communication Coach

Jack's supervisor asked him to put together a new plan for orienting new nurses to the unit. Jack, a Baby Boomer preceptor, included other Baby Boomers on his team, thinking that their experience would strengthen the plan. When Jack presented the plan to the staff members, he had to field questions from Gen Yers as to why there weren't more online options, and Gen Xers pointed out several practical flaws. Jack went back to the drawing board with a new team and revised the plan, which was well received by the staff.

Lesson: Jack learned that each generation brings a unique perspective to problem solving. Veterans tend to be logical thinkers; Baby Boomers excel at teams and applying their experience; Gen Yers like to participate and are technology oriented; and Gen Xers are pragmatic, skeptical, and outcomes-oriented—and often identify flaws in plans, as Jack found out.

How do different generations approach teamwork?

Baby Boomers tend to focus on building consensus, whereas Gen Yers see a lack of consensus as helpful for moving the reasoning process to a "higher level" (Glennon, 2009). Gen X has a self-reliant attitude (I'll do it myself) that may make Gen Yers feel excluded. It's important that team members respect all points of view.

What is the best match for preceptors among generations?

Some experts recommend matching preceptors and preceptees by age. However, in nursing, that solution is often unrealistic because of imbalances in experiences and group numbers. You may find that

Gen Y and Baby Boomers make a good fit. Both are positive and like teams and group discussion. Additionally, Baby Boomers like to teach and Gen Yers like to learn (Erickson 2008). Keep in mind that Gen Yers expect the most coaching and mentoring compared to other generations (Sherman, 2006).

It has often been said that people from Gen Y are self-centered. What's the truth?

It's a myth that Gen Y is self-centered. More than 80% of Gen Yers have volunteered in the past year and trust a company more if it is socially or environmentally responsible (Erickson, 2008). In many cases, volunteerism has been part of their school curriculum, so they have a strong community orientation (Winograd & Hais, 2008).

TIP

Gen Y is the most racially diverse generation: 61% are white, 17% Hispanic, 15% African American, and 4% Asian. This helps them to excel in diverse groups. They also have a global perspective that other generations can tap into.
(Erickson, 2008)

"In case you're worried about what's going to become of the younger generation, it's going to grow up and start worrying about the younger generation."

—Roger Allen

Supporting Motivation

What are some ways to manage Gen Yers?

Here are a few strategies (Stanton Smith, 2008):

* Let them have fun and be as independent as possible

* Realize they want to work with their friends

* Mentor, don't micromanage

* Provide rationales

* Respect what they bring

* Challenge them with variety

* Lead as an experienced colleague, not a boss

TIP

Don't assume which generation is happiest at work. According to a Canadian study, Baby Boomers are significantly more satisfied with work than Gen X or Gen Y (Wilson et al, 2008).

How can managers motivate staff from differing generations?

The best way is to ask what motivates them, but here are some general guidelines for each generation:

* Veterans: A job well done, personal touches

* Baby Boomers: Money, title, recognition, perks

* Gen X: Freedom, paid time off, exciting projects

* Gen Y: Meaningful work

See Table 8.4 for specific suggestions.

8.4 — Motivation strategies

Generation	Suggestions
Veterans	Show respect and interest; acknowledge experience
Baby Boomers	Give recognition for work; give positive feedback when goal is reached
Gen X	Give freedom when possible; remember they will work around the rules if they don't like them
Gen Y	Support them in their goals; provide strong mentorship and guidance

(Siela, 2006; Lower, 2007)

"If you want happiness for a lifetime, help the next generation."

–Chinese Proverb

✔ Checklist

Generational Communication

❑ Do I understand the differences of the four generations?

❑ Do I consider the values of my colleagues from different generations?

❑ Have I considered what I have in common with the other person?

❑ Am I ready to create an intergenerational team?

❑ Do I tailor my management and communication style to each generation?

❑ Am I prepared to use each generation's preferred technology for communicating?

❑ Am I mindful that each person is an individual?

Frequently Asked Questions

 How can I better understand how the people I work with fit into the generation model?

A fun activity for a staff meeting or even an informal lunch can be to present the generational differences, ask where each member falls (without getting age specific), and then discuss what they agree and disagree with in the description.

 Isn't all this talk about generations just stereotyping?

Generational differences are not hard-and-fast rules. They are simply tools to help us better understand one another. As Karlene Kerfoot, vice president and chief clinical officer for Aurora Health Care, says, "Our oldest nurse working in a direct caregiver position is 84, and she works in a unit with every generational group. It's one of the highest-functioning units because they have a synergized team that has concentrated on valuing differences" (Personal Communication, 2009).

 I try to give my new Gen Y coworker plenty of feedback, but my Gen X coworkers think I'm coddling him. What should I do?

Gen X workers tend to believe that frustration and failure build character and are a natural part of life (Glennon, 2009). Explain that Gen Y comes from an era when they received much attention from parents and teachers and, therefore, need a bit more "attention" at work.

I'm a nurse executive. Is there going to be anyone from future generations who will take my place?

Succession planning is a challenge in an era when younger generations value work-life balance. It's vital to integrate leadership development into the organization setting, similar to how Kristine Campbell, RN, executive director of the Oregon Center for Nursing in Portland, says the military integrates such development into its system. Campbell, a retired brigadier general from the U.S. Army Reserves, says because the Army has to hire from within, "it starts leadership development from the day you start and invests in you all along," something that hospitals often fail to do (Rollins, 2008).

 What are the most common misunderstandings in intergenerational teams?

Tammy Erickson, *Harvard Business Review* blog, says generational conflict is typically related to four team activities:

1. Choosing where and when to work

2. Communicating among team members

3. Getting together

4. Finding information or learning new things (2009).

You can use your skills to address the communication issues.

 What other strategies can I use to teach Gen Yers?

Pardue and Morgan (2008) recommend teachers accept multitasking and incorporate text, graphics, sound, and kinesthetic learning into their teaching. Active questioning, group work, multimedia, and hands-on activities are techniques preceptors can adapt from academic teachers.

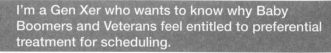

 I'm a Gen Xer who wants to know why Baby Boomers and Veterans feel entitled to preferential treatment for scheduling.

Older workers believe they have "paid their dues" and deserve special treatment. Younger workers do not see the need to wait in line. One way to deal with this is to put together an intergenerational team to develop fair scheduling practices (Hannon 2009).

 My organization has banned social networking at work. How can I change their minds?

Use facts to show that workers aren't abusing social networking. One study reported that although 59% of Gen Y and Gen X use social technologies at home, only 14% do so in the workplace (Information Outlook, 2009). This strategy may also affect recruitment. In an Australian study, nearly half the employees who use MySpace and Facebook during work hours would turn down a job offer from a potential employer that banned such sites. And, as Phil Baumann, RN, who blogs about technology said, "People are going to socialize (whether or not they have access to social media). It's a natural, healthy part of the work environment" (Saver, 2010).

How am I supposed to know how everyone likes to communicate?

Ask.

TAKE-AWAY TIPS

✔ **Different generations have different values and preferred ways of communicating.**

✔ **Ask people how they prefer to communicate and what motivates them.**

✔ **Don't generalize generational descriptions; each person is an individual.**

✔ **Understand that each generation makes a valuable contribution to the workplace.**

9

*

Social Media

Do you:

Wonder how to open a Twitter profile?

Know how a blog differs from a website?

Ever get a Facebook "friend" request that you don't want to accept?

Know how to determine whether a social network will work for you?

Wonder if LinkedIn can enhance your career prospects?

Know if your organization has an internal or external blog?

Understanding and utilizing social media can be a powerful tool for communicating and building relationships. Using social media properly and knowing who can access your information will help you decide what tools to use and what to post. New tools are only as good as your ability to use them; therefore, you must be open to learning something new. By participating and being part of the action, social media can make a difference in your personal and professional life.

Social Media Explained

What exactly is social media?

Social media is a term used to describe any kind of consumer-generated media or content that can be uploaded to the Internet and easily located and shared. The media can be in many forms, such as text, images, audio, or video.

What are some examples of social media formats on the Internet or other digital platforms?

* Written forms of communication can be found on blogs, web forums, message boards, e-mail discussion lists, wikis, etc.

* Photographs can be displayed as images on image-sharing sites, such as Flickr.

* Audio broadcasts can be created as podcasts.

* Video clips can be uploaded to YouTube or other video sharing sites (Berkman, 2008).

TIP

With all forms of communication, play nice, say "thank you," and foster relationships.

Why is it important for health care professionals to get involved with social media?

The various forms of social media are powerful communication tools. A key aspect of health care is communication. Social media is also a great source of free information.

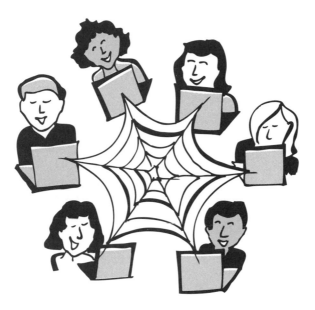

Social Networking Profiles

What is the main purpose of social networking sites?

They are online meeting places. They make it easy to create a profile, which in turn makes it easy to make friends in a social context or make business contacts in a professional context. Sites such as Facebook, MySpace, and LinkedIn make it easy for people to keep in touch with the people and organizations they are interested in. They also are a great way to maintain relationships. This is especially important today because young people are prone to move around the country (and sometimes around the world).

How many adults have a profile on an online networking site?

According to a January 2009 Pew study, 35% of adults and 75% of 18-24 year olds have an online profile (Saver, 2010).

Can you provide a brief description of Facebook?

The fundamental function of Facebook is sharing information between "friends." Friends are people who have agreed to communicate and allow each other some level of access to personal information and activities. Members connect by a "friend request" process. Friends can also be found by letting Facebook search your e-mail addresses or by looking at the lists of other friends' friends.

Your profile can remain private until you approve someone as your Facebook friend. Or, your profile can be public, meaning anyone can find you and view your profile, pictures, and so on.

Facebook is one of the fastest-growing social networking sites (if not the fastest). Anyone can join Facebook and find and connect with existing or new contacts (friends). They are alerted by a news feed to activities their "friends" have been doing (for example, Tim placed second in a triathlon).

Communication Coach

Jim, age 60, recently joined Facebook. He was delighted when he was connected to a former player from a basketball team he coached. The young woman said how much she enjoyed basketball because she (and everyone on the team) played in every game. The former coach was delighted. Although his belief and practice in playing all members of the team was often criticized by the parents of the better players, he thought it was the right thing to do.

Lesson: Facebook connections can share that someone made a difference.

What is typically in a Facebook profile?

Members usually include a picture and some basic information (such as where they live, workplace, education, hobbies, interests, etc).

Can people connect to groups on Facebook?

Yes. Groups are a great way to connect and inform interested people. All users can create groups. They can have open membership (anyone can join) or keep the group closed (invitation only).

Wasn't Facebook just for students at one time?

Yes. When Facebook started, it was available only to college students. Prior to September 2006, users needed an e-mail address ending in .edu to qualify for an account. When Facebook was opened to nonstudents, its popularity exploded, with traffic doubling in less than a year (Scott, 2009).

Communication Coach

A former factory worker was receiving disability payments because she was incapacitated by a work-related injury. Her disability payments were stopped when pictures on her Facebook account showed her partying at a bar in the Bahamas.

Lesson: Be careful of what you put on Facebook. You never know who will share your information. Privacy settings are essential for photo albums.

How is MySpace different than Facebook?

MySpace was originally targeted to teens and young people. Although MySpace is still predominately populated by young people, adults also participate in this site. One media expert found that Facebook has been attracting more middle- and upper-class and college-educated users, whereas MySpace has more working class users (Berkman, 2008).

MySpace also allows for more personalization through customization of your profile page. For example, you can change the colors, post background pictures, add music, and so on. Musicians like this site. You can check an artist's page, download music, and see tour dates.

Why are professionals joining LinkedIn?

LinkedIn is an online professional contact database that allows members to create a profile and link their profiles with connections they know and trust. Based on recommendations from their network, members can use LinkedIn to find jobs and business opportunities.

LinkedIn helps people keep in touch with people they have worked with in the past, even if they have changed jobs or switched positions. LinkedIn can network the right person with the right contact at the right time.

Communication Coach

When JB moved to the Philadelphia area, he updated his LinkedIn profile with his new address. As a result, three contacts reached out to him to discuss his new job activities and offer their assistance. Without LinkedIn, he would not have reconnected with these contacts.

Lesson: When mutually relevant information is displayed on a social networking site, people can reconnect and provide support.

How can employers use LinkedIn?

LinkedIn can help employers find employees and get background information on them. For example, organizations can find out where the candidates worked before and who they worked for.

People can also research potential employers or interviewers on LinkedIn. Be careful, however, because people can check who has been viewing their profile. Comparatively, Facebook claims it is impossible to determine who has been looking at your profile.

What are the different levels of connection of LinkedIn?

Levels of connection are based on how well you know others. For example:

* Primary or first connections: people whom the user knows directly and to whom they are immediately linked. This means they can be viewed and contacted at any time.

* Second-degree connections: These are contacts known by the people you know.

* Third-degree connections: These are contacts of your second-degree connections.

* Remaining degree connections continue as such.

Your possible list of connections increases exponentially based on the connections of your connections. Through your connections, you increase the likelihood that someone you know can facilitate a desired introduction or connection for you.

Communication Coach

A book author (Edward) wanted to interview the CEO of a major company. A LinkedIn search of the CEO (Mark) showed that he was three degrees separated from the author. The chain of acquaintances revealed a direct contact named Doug, who was directly connected to someone named Steve, with whom the author had worked. Steve went to college with Mark! Within 30 minutes of contacting Doug, Ed received a call from Mark.

Lesson: Connecting with someone via a warm connection is easier than a cold call. That, and belonging to a trusted network, is the power of LinkedIn.

How can you be sure your social networking sites are beneficial for career advancement?

Make certain that your online information leaves no opportunity for misinterpretation. Potential employers can view your profile. Many employers prescreen applicants using social media sites. Inappropriate photos and comments can disqualify job candidates (Liburdi, 2008).

What are some recommendations for getting the most from social networking sites?

See Table 9.1 for some do's and don'ts (Liburdi, 2008):

9.1	Do's and Don'ts for Social Networking Sites
DO	**DON'T**
Evaluate your profile and postings.	Share too much personal information online.
Google your name and see what results appear.	Post daily schedules, social dates, phone numbers, hotel room numbers, or home addresses.
Post accomplishments and interests.	Post incriminating photos or videos online.
Use your privacy settings to control who has access to your information	Trust all users on social networking sites.
Tell your friends not to use your photos or videos without permission.	Post anything you would feel uncomfortable with a potential employer reading on your profile.

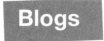

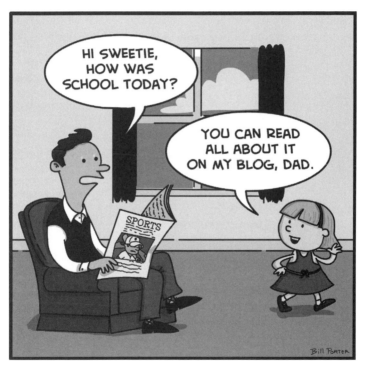

© 2007 Bill Porter.

"Eventually, most businesses will use blogs to communicate with customers, suppliers, and employers because it's two-way and more satisfying."

–Bill Gates

What is a blog, and where did the term "blog" come from?

Blog comes from "Weblog," which is an online journal. A blog is a website maintained by a person with regular entries or posts that include thoughts, ideas, and commentaries. Photos, graphics, audio, and video can be part of the posts. Blogs can provide news and content on a specific subject or can operate as personal journals (Safko & Brake, 2009).

Blog entries are displayed in reverse chronological order. The most recent post appears at the top of the page.

How are blogs different than websites?

Blogs are more engaging than static websites. Here are some differences:

* Blogs are interactive.

* Blogs are written in a conversational tone.

* Blogs are created using instant software. No tech expertise is needed.

* Blogs can alert readers whenever something new is added without e-mail.

* Blogs are frequently updated.

* Blogs get higher rankings in search engines than static websites.

* Blogs are a form of viral marketing.
  (Weil, 2006)

What is the blogosphere?

Blogosphere refers to all the blogs on the Internet and bloghood refers to a collection of blogs in the same geographical area.

What kind of software is needed to start a blog?

Choices for setting up a blog include WordPress.com and
Blogger.com among numerous others. These are free options.
A blog is easy to create and can be up and running in a few minutes.
Other software with monthly fees is available for purchase.

How often do bloggers post content on their blogs?

This varies. For example, bloggers can post daily, several times a
week, once a week, and so on.

Don't let a month-old post sit on your blog without
an explanation. If you need to take a break from
blogging, post a reason for your hiatus and tell
your readers when to expect you back (Weil,
2006).

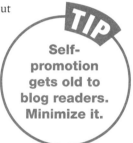

Self-promotion gets old to blog readers. Minimize it.

Maintaining a blog requires dedication and
effort. The time you invest in blogging is related to the purpose of the blog and your time
priorities.

Is there a recommended length for a blog post?

Lengths vary. But for the most part, posts are short. Longer posts
are okay now and then, but not on a regular basis. A good goal is
under 1000 words (Holtz & Demopoulos, 2006).

How do blog readers know when you post a new entry?

An essential feature of a blog is an RSS (Really Simple Syndication)
feed or web feed. An RSS feed lets readers subscribe to a blog via an
RSS newsreader, such as NewsGator, iGoogle, or Bloglines, among
others, and receive an automatic update every time content is added.
Because e-mail is not needed, the updates are not blocked by spam
filters or lost in a clogged Inbox (Weil, 2006).

"The tipping point for 'wait and see' (about blogs) is swinging, like a metronome, toward 'better do something now.'"

–Debbie Weil

What are some tips for becoming an effective blogger?

Here are some suggestions by David Risley, who has been blogging for a living for many years (Safko & Brake, 2009):

* Post often

* Use catchy blog post titles

* Ask open-ended questions

* Comment on other blogs

* Use images in your posts

* Offer unique and/or helpful information

* Link to other related blog posts

* Focus your blog around a certain mission or theme

* Be yourself and show your personality on your blog

* Write like you are talking to people

* Link to your social profiles on your blog

* Read other blogs

How much information should the blog include about the author?

When people visit a site, they want background information on the author. It is a good idea to include an "about" page that includes a photo, biography, affiliations, and information about the blogger.

What are some of the key features of blogs?

Here are some of the most important features that have contributed to its popularity:

* Blogs allow for two-way communication.

* Readers can interact with the author through comments.

* Starting a blog is simple and easy.

* By providing good content, blogs can position the blogger as an industry leader.

* Blogs generate a higher ranking on Google.

* Adding a post to a blog is as easy as sending an e-mail.

TIP

Blogging is a social activity. Be proactive in your niche and accessible to your readers.

Can blogs increase traffic to a website?

Yes. Search engines love blogs. They list their latest posts in top positions—ahead of websites (Scott, 2009).

"Use this mnemonic: BLOG stands for Better Listings on Google."

–Rick Bruner

How are comments handled on a blog?

Blogging software allows for several options. One option is to not allow comments, but that eliminates a popular feature of blogs. You can opt for open comments where people can write comments that are not subject to your approval or you can opt to approve comments before they appear on the blog.

Many bloggers use the approval option to avoid inappropriate comments. However, you should allow comments from people who disagree with you because healthy debate is an indicator of a well-read blog (Scott, 2009). If only rosy comments are posted, credibility suffers.

Communication Coach

In a *60 Minutes* broadcast in September 2004, documents were presented that were critical of President George W. Bush's service in the National Guard. The documents were presented as authentic, but had not been properly authenticated. When bloggers questioned the authenticity of the documents, Dan Rather dismissed the bloggers as a bunch of geeks in pajamas. Ignoring the bloggers cost him his job. Had he taken them seriously and investigated the documents, he would have concluded the documents were false.

Lesson: Do not dismiss the opinions of bloggers and underestimate their influence (Scott, 2009).

"Blogs are often misperceived by people who don't read them."

–David M. Scott

Are blogs used mainly for personal or business reasons?

They are used for both. A person can have both types of blogs. Business blogs can be used for internal communication with employees or can be open to the public.

When did businesses begin to take blogs seriously?

In the May 2, 2005 issue of *Business Week*, the journal stated that blogging is here to stay as a business consideration (Holtz & Demopoulos, 2006). Companies that publish blogs can help repair the public's damaged perception of corporate America by providing authenticity, transparency, and immediacy (Weil, 2006).

How are businesses using blogs?

Listed below are some of the ways blogs are being used in business:

* For company leaders to communicate with customers

* For employees to communicate with customers

* For employers to share information with employees via intranet

* For customers to provide unsolicited feedback (preferences, complaints, suggestions)

* To engage customers

* For branding, marketing, and sales

* To keep customers updated on product issues

* To attract new business

* To recruit the best employees

* To provide timely updates to the public in a crisis

* To report to a constituency audience on company policy

* To advocate specific issues (such as health care)

How can companies use blogs inside their organizations?

Blogs can be mounted on an intranet and made available to employees. They can transform a static, one-way, top-down intranet into a dynamic, interactive collaboration tool. Intranet blogs facilitate knowledge transfer and provide a foundation for institutional memory. Blogs lend themselves to internal uses within a company. Here are some general categories:

* Project blogs (journals and team blogs)

* News blogs (birthdays, babies, achievements, parties, etc.)

* Customer and competitor blogs (feedback from customers and information about competitors)

* Interdepartmental team blogs (connect people who don't work in same department)

* Individual employee blogs (speeds transfer of knowledge through the organization)

* Department blogs (authored by the manager or by the employees)

* CEO blogs (explain decisions, ask for ideas)
  (Holtz & Demopoulos, 2006).

Is it okay to pitch products or sales on your blog?

No. That will turn off your readers. If you have products to sell, it is better to have a link to your website and shopping cart.

Most social media sites are promoting themselves in one form or another. The key is to create demand for your services through demonstrated expertise, relevance, and information versus solicitation. Pull the audience in versus pushing them.

Are there different kinds of blogs?

Yes, there are many different blog types. Here are some examples (Safko & Brake, 2009):

* Qlog: a question blog where readers submit questions

* Vlog: a blog site that posts video

* Linklogs: blogs that post links to other blogs

* Tumbleblogs: blogs that feature shorter posts and mixed media

* Blawgs: blogs about legal issues

How does a reader find a blog for a particular topic or area of interest?

Some good places to start include Google, Yahoo!, BlogSearch, and Technorati. Technorati (www.technorati.com) is the most popular blog search site and the most comprehensive source of information on the blogosphere (Safko & Brake, 2009).

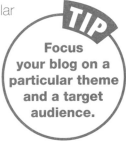

Focus your blog on a particular theme and a target audience.

How do you know if a blog is credible?

Don't believe everything you read. Blogs build credibility the same way as any other source of information. Blogs need to earn your trust.

How quickly is the number of blogs increasing?

The best way to answer this is to give an example (Berkman, 2008). According to Technorati, there were 9 million blogs in 2005; 32 million blogs in 2006; and over 80 million blogs in 2007.

What are "blooks?"

Many bloggers have published books based on their original blog posts. They are called "blooks." Some examples include *The Clandestine Diary of an Ordinary Iraqi* by Salam Pax and *Diary of a Dysfunctional Flight Attendant: The Queen of the Sky Blog* by Ellen Simonetti.

Communication Coach

Starbucks has a blog-based website that facilitates conversations among employees and customers. When a barista from Minnesota got fired for trying to unionize employees, he was reinstated, most likely because of the coverage the event received on the Starbucks blog.

Lesson: Employee and customer opinion can have an impact on a business (Safko & Brake, 2009).

Twitter

What is Twitter, and why has it gotten so popular?

Twitter's simplicity is the reason for its success and popularity. It is a microblogging application that asks the question: "What are you doing?" Users can post status updates or "tweets" as often as they like via mobile phone, instant messaging, or a web browser. Posts must be under 140 characters. They are displayed on the user's technology of choice (text-messaging cell phone, website, PDA, Twitter website, e-mail, Facebook, etc.).

What is the point of responding to the question "What are you doing?"

There is no point if you respond with, "I am eating my breakfast." However, when used strategically, Twitter can connect with others, build brands, provide project updates, and promote services or products. People use Twitter to keep their "followers" (people who subscribe to their Twitter feed) updated about their lives. Users can follow the Twitter updates of anyone they choose (such as, family, colleagues, book authors, athletes, and movie stars).

What are some basic terms associated with Twitter?

Here are some of the basics about Twitter, the most prevalent micro-blogging technology (Safko & Brake, 2009):

* A "Twitterer" is a person using Twitter to send "tweets" or posts.

* A "Tweet" is a text message or post sent from one Twitterer to another.

* The Tweeting community is called the "Twitosphere."

* When you hit Send, the tweet is out there. A regretted tweet is called a "MisTweet."

How is Twitter different than blogging or sending an e-mail?

Because of the constraint on the size of a tweet, people use Twitter to update their networks with information that is more concise than a blog post and more casual than an e-mail (Scott, 2009).

Communication Coach

A business traveler went on-line to find a hotel room in NYC and was disappointed that no rooms in midtown were available. He sent a tweet to his network and immediately heard from a number of people with suggestions. Within minutes, he had reservations at a boutique hotel in midtown Manhattan.

Lesson: Twitter can be a powerful personal and professional network. If you invest in your relationships, it can work in your favor when needed (Scott, 2009).

What are some guidelines for using Twitter?

Here are some tips for effective use of this new communication tool:

* Use @replies to start conversations

* Re-tweet (RT) posts you find interesting

* Be part of the conversation rather than just watching the feed go by

* Upload a photo of yourself to distinguish you from spammers and make you feel "real"

* Be gracious to those who promote your tweets

* Thank fans for passing along your praises and return the favor

* Keep the content a mix of information, thoughts, recommendations, and resources

* Ask questions, provide answers, share news, provide links, and use pithy sayings

* Minimize promotion of yourself or your organization

What do you do if you no longer want to follow someone on Twitter?

You can simply "Un-Follow" that person. This is the power of permission-based marketing. You choose who is allowed to market and communicate with you. When someone you are following ceases to deliver relevant, "What's in it for me?" content, that's the time to opt out of following that person (Safko & Brake, 2009).

What should you do if Twitter loses its appeal or becomes overwhelming?

Back off and Un-Follow. Moderation is the key.

How can you use Twitter as a networking tool?

When you get your account up and running, here are some ideas to build your network:

TIP

Don't tweet anything you would not want to see on the front page of a newspaper or famous website.

* Follow interesting people. Use a Twitter search, such as Twellow (www.twellow.com), to search by name, profession, or interest. Twellow is the Yellow Pages directory of Twitter.

* Have Twitter search your Google, Yahoo!, and AOL accounts.

* Use Twellowhood (www.twellowhood.com) to find twitters in a certain area.

* Follow conversations for a period and then join in.

* If you are interested in connecting with someone, retweet some of their messages before introducing yourself.

* Post your profile on Twitter and link to your website or blog.

* Use Twhirl (www.twhirl.org) to cross-post your updates to sites like Facebook and LinkedIn.

* Send tweets via your mobile phone with Tiny Twitter (www.tinytwitter.com).

* Feed your blog to your Twitter account by using TwitterFeed (http://twitterfeed.com).

* Deliver your tweets directly to your blog with LoudTwitter (www.loudtwitter.com).

* Create connections. Do not spam.

Communication Coach

Donna planned to attend the AORN national conference in Seattle. Before leaving for the conference, she posted a tweet saying when she would be in Seattle. She got a tweet back from someone else planning to be at the same conference. They ended up meeting in person.

Lesson: Twitter can facilitate face-to-face meetings that would not have occurred otherwise.

Can you give some examples of how businesses use Twitter?

Because of the broadcast-like structure of microblogging, thousands of people can receive the information instantaneously (Scott, 2009). Here are some examples (Safko & Brake, 2009):

* Southwest Airlines regularly tweets as a customer service tool.

* Whole Foods Market uses Twitter to provide product information.

* The Los Angeles Fire Department uses Twitter to get up-to-the-second information on where fires are breaking out and where people are trapped.

* NASA uses Twitter to provide updates on space shuttle missions.

* News outlets, such as the BBC, use Twitter to disseminate breaking news.

* Several 2008 U.S. Presidential campaigns used Twitter as a publicity mechanism.

How can you create a Twitter account? Is there a cost?

Go to www.twitter.com. This is a free social networking service.

Is Twitter the only microblogging platform?

No. Twitter is the most popular but there are many others. Examples include Jaiku, PlaceShout, Plurk, Yammer, Prologue, and Dodgeball.

Forums

What is the status of forums and discussion groups?

Before blogs emerged in the mid 1990s, Internet users could have discussions many places online. Examples include forums, bulletin boards, USENET groups, and ListServs. These discussion groups contain a goldmine of valuable opinion and discussion. However, they tend to be overlooked today by amateur and professional researchers (Berkman, 2008).

Why are these forums and discussion groups overlooked today?

Here are three reasons (Berkman, 2008):

* Their search engines are not as well known as Google and Technorati.

* These older formats are associated with undesirable types of online communication, such as spam and irrelevant comments.

* These older formats seem outdated with today's interactive two-way mediums.

How do social networking sites differ from the organizational focus of older forums and discussion groups?

Online communities, such as USENET and discussion groups, were structured around topics. Comparatively, social network sites are primarily organized with individuals at the center of their own communities (Boyd & Ellison, 2007).

Commonly Used Social Media Terms

Del.icio.us: The most popular social bookmarking site.

Flickr: A popular site for sharing and tagging images.

ListServ: The very first e-mail list discussion software.

Mashup: A combination of digital information, data, or programs to create something new.

News feed: Frequently updated content typically created in the RSS (see below) standard so Internet users with a news reader can receive regular updates.

News reader: Software that lets users collect and read RSS news feeds from frequently updated sites.

Podcast: An online radio show that can be listened to on a PC, cell phone, or media player (such as an iPod).

Post: An entry on a blog or the act of posting a blog.

RSS: This is an acronym for Really Simple Syndication (or Rich Site Summary), a content syndication format used to categorize content and deliver dynamic web content without the need for visiting each site. For example, RSS is used by bloggers to distribute their latest postings. RSS also provides notification to users whenever a blog or other frequently updated site they follow has published new content.

Social bookmarking: The way web users save and share URLs. The most popular is del.icio.us.

Tagging: Adding a word or phrase to any form of content (such as text or audio) to identify and describe it.

Technorati: A search engine for indexing blogs and other consumer-generated media.

USENET: The original Internet-based online discussion groups. These discussion groups preceded the Web.

Wiki: A software program that permits multiple people to remotely collaborate on the same document and make changes without anyone's consent. The most popular is the online encyclopedia, Wikipedia.

YouTube: A site owned by Google where anyone can upload digital videos and watch videos made by others.

✔ *Checklist*

Social Media

- ❏ Am I open to learning about these new forms of technology?

- ❏ Do I understand the difference between a blog and a website?

- ❏ Can I see how different forms of social media could impact my work setting?

- ❏ Did I Google myself and examine the results?

- ❏ Do I have a plan for exploring and trying some form of social media?

- ❏ Can I see the connection between social networking in the offline world and online social network sites?

❑ Did I discover any technology that could help my organization develop trust and cultivate customer relationships?

❑ Can I determine ways that blogging could enhance health care communication in my setting?

❑ Am I aware of the potential career impact of posting inappropriate things on a Facebook account?

❑ Can I describe different ways that businesses are using Twitter?

Frequently Asked Questions

What should you do if your boss sends you a Facebook friend request that you don't want to accept?

You are under no obligation to accept. If you do accept, be sure to check your privacy settings so your boss only sees the information you want him or her to view.

Do you need to give an explanation if you de-friend someone on Facebook?

No. However, do so if you think it would be polite to offer an explanation. Facebook doesn't send out a notification when someone is de-friended. So, the person may never know. They just stop receiving your updates in their news feed.

Can spam filters intercept and block blogs?

No. Unlike e-mail, blogs skirt around spam filters. This is one reason that many people with electronic newsletters are switching to blogs. Blogs use an RSS feed instead of e-mail, which can be blocked by spam filters.

How can companies ensure that employee blogs remain focused on business and work?

By articulating and communicating an internal blogging policy. However, because work is social, it is a good idea for these internal blogs to have some fun posts and some non-work-related content (Holtz & Demopoulos, 2006).

 How much does a non-techie need to know about the technical features of blogging?

Not much. Blogging software is user-friendly. If you can send an e-mail, you can compose and publish a blog (Weil, 2006).

 What is Web 2.0?

This is a term used to describe the evolution of the web from its original static, one-way form (Web 1.0) to its more interactive two-way format. Web 2.0 is sometimes used to refer to more user-friendly design principles and the automatic updating of content without downloading a new, static web page.

 Is it okay to blog or write on Facebook about patients you take care of as long as you don't mention any names?

Be careful here. Any information about a patient that allows another person to recognize the patient is a breach of confidentiality. Think of how someone would feel if they could identify themselves or a family member on your Facebook page or blog. A breach of confidentiality could result in job termination, fines, penalties, and jail time.

TAKE-AWAY TIPS

✓ **Social media is redefining the way people communicate and do business.**

✓ **Modern technology hasn't eliminated the need to meet at the water cooler, but it has increased the amount of information available to share (Safko & Brake).**

✓ **Social media is designed to be easily shared, collaborative, openly accessible, and easily retrievable by others (Berkman, 2008).**

✓ **Blogs facilitate conversation, and conversation builds trust.**

✓ **Blogs provide experts and wannabes with an easy way to make their voices heard.**

✓ **It takes a long time to develop trust and build a following on Twitter. It takes one Tweet to alienate all of your followers.**

✓ **The importance of social media is undervalued by those who do not understand them.**

10

*

Cross-Cultural Communication

Do you:

Know how negotiating styles can vary from culture to culture?

Wonder if you offended an international colleague with a joke?

Consider cultural differences in perceptions of time?

Know what it means when your colleague nods his head?

Avoid gestures that may offend international colleagues?

Translate "yes" and "no" responses with care?

Know how to demonstrate respect in formal cultures?

Effective communication is difficult under the best of circumstances. However, cross-cultural factors create the potential for increased communication problems because of the culture gap between you and your international colleagues. Misunderstandings arise when people assume their own beliefs, attitudes, and behaviors are normal. In many cases, people are unaware that others may look at the world from a completely different perspective.

This chapter helps you learn what other cultures value and what lies behind their beliefs. Note that this chapter uses generalizations about cultural differences. Because there are variations within every culture, you need further information to determine whether the generalization applies to a particular person. People are unique and should not be stereotyped.

"Manners must adorn knowledge and smooth its way through the world."

–Lord Chesterfield

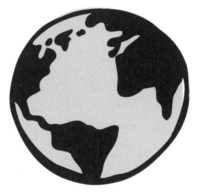

Rigid-Time and Fluid-Time Cultures

How do time and scheduling impact international business relationships?

People look at time and scheduling differently in different parts of the world. In rigid-time societies, punctuality is critical. Schedules and agendas are fixed, and meetings are rarely interrupted. These clock-obsessed cultures are often called monochronic. Time is linear, sequential, and can be cut into blocks. People are judged by how well they control their time.

Comparatively, fluid-time cultures place less emphasis on punctuality and deadlines. These cultures are often called polychronic. Time is circular and a servant, not a master. How people manage relationships is more important than how they manage their time. People may show up late for events and not feel obliged to apologize. These cultures value loose scheduling and meetings where several meetings-within-meetings may be taking place simultaneously. Ending an ongoing meeting just because another meeting is scheduled is considered rude (Gesteland, 2005).

What are some examples of monochronic cultures?

Examples include North America, Nordic and Germanic Europe, and Japan.

What are some examples of polychronic cultures?

Examples include the Arabic-speaking countries, Africa, Southeast Asia, and Latin America.

> **TIP**
> There is a big difference in the meaning of "a little late" in a monochronic and a polychronic culture.

Can orientations to time vary within a country?

Yes. Europe is a good example. The northern part of the continent values punctuality. For example, punctuality is expected in Germany. In the southern part of Europe, time becomes more fluid. As an example, in Naples, being 45 minutes late for a business meeting is not unusual (Gesteland, 2005).

Communication Coach

A Malaysian businesswoman flew to the United States for a meeting scheduled for 10 AM on a Tuesday morning in Philadelphia. She arrived in Philadelphia late Monday evening and overslept the next morning. By the time she arrived at the meeting location, it was 2 PM and the company could not rearrange their scheduled afternoon meetings to accommodate her. She thought the Americans were rude.

Lesson: Visitors to foreign countries need to consider and respect the cultural time orientation of the country where they are doing business. Visitors are expected to acquiesce to local customs.

What are some guidelines for dealing with people in monochronic cultures?

Here are some tips to use in rigid-time cultures:

* Make appointments well in advance. This shows you are in control of your time.

* Send meeting agendas in advance.

* Arrive on time.

* Start your meeting on time. If visitors are kept waiting, they may think you are disorganized and you may lose their respect or trust. If there is an unavoidable delay, explain the reason and apologize.

* Keep to your agenda, schedule, and deadline.

* Interrupt if you do not understand something. Waiting until the end of the meeting before admitting this is considered wasting time.

* Be upfront with bad news. Withholding bad news is considered dishonest or deceitful (Carte & Fox, 2004).

What are some guidelines for dealing with people in polychronic cultures?

Here are some tips to use in fluid-time cultures:

* Fix appointments at short notice. Don't be surprised if meeting times need to change at the last minute.

* Allow plenty of time between appointments.

* Be prepared to be kept waiting. Bring a brief case with things to read. Don't keep looking at your watch and don't complain. Use the time to chat to the receptionist or other visitors.

* Try to set an agenda at the beginning of the meeting. Allow participants to meander with the discussion.

* Avoid rushing meetings.

* Don't bind yourself to self-imposed deadlines. Don't quickly wind up the discussion to catch a plane home.

* If there is bad news, try to soften it. Spend a little time preparing others for what you are going to say (Carte & Fox, 2004).

What is the meaning of a future or present-time orientation?

Most middle-class Americans tend to be future oriented in their perception of time. They tend to defer gratification of personal pleasure until meeting a future goal, such as advanced education. These individuals tend to structure time rigidly. They adhere to a time schedule in their work and social activities.

TIP

If you are invited to a party or a dinner, find out what time you are actually expected to arrive.

For present-oriented individuals, the present takes precedence over the future and the past. These individuals do not adhere to a strict time schedule. What is happening in the present may be more important than a future appointment. For this reason, they may be late for appointments (Giger & Davidhizar, 2008).

Emotionally Expressive and Emotionally Reserved Cultures

How does emotion affect communication in different cultures?

Varying degrees of expressiveness can cause problems with international communications. Some cultures are very reserved or restrained with their emotions. Other cultures are very expressive with loud voices, animated facial expressions, and numerous hand gestures.

What are some examples of very reserved cultures?

Examples include East and Southeast Asia and Nordic and Germanic Europe. In these cultures, a loud and exuberant communication style would cause problems.

TIP

When in doubt, respectfully ask. This shows interest and will improve communication.

What are some examples of very expressive cultures?

Countries in the Mediterranean region and Latin America are good examples. In these cultures, a soft voice, an expressionless face, and little or no gesturing would complicate communication.

How do reserved and expressive cultures respond to periods of silence?

Expressive people tend to feel uncomfortable with silence in a conversation. After a few seconds of silence, they feel compelled to say something or anything to break the silence. The loquacity of expressive people can irritate people from reserved cultures.

People from reserved cultures do not feel the need to constantly babble during a conversation. They feel comfortable with periods of silence. For example, the Japanese value the space between the spoken words as much as the words.

How do reserved and expressive cultures respond to interruptions during a conversation?

Expressive people regard interruptions as a normal part of conversation. Comparatively, reserved cultures consider interruptions rude. Problems can occur unless both communicators know about this cultural difference. For example, Middle Easterners may think the Japanese are indecisive or at loss for words, while the Japanese may find Middle Easterners insulting and rude (Gesteland, 2005).

Communication Coach

Jane was a very successful director of a trade association in Singapore. As an outgoing and enthusiastic American, she was delighted when she was asked to chair a women's conference in Thailand. Her friends and colleagues warned her that Thai women tend to be shy in public. During the first session, Jane was thrilled when several Thai participants quietly offered some comments. She profusely thanked them in a loud and exuberant voice so that all attendees could hear. When the meeting continued, there was no more input from the audience. After the meeting, the two women who had spoken in the morning tearfully asked Jane why she was angry with them.

Lesson: Jane should have listened to the advice of her colleagues. The Thai culture is a very reserved culture.

Formal and Informal Cultures

How does the formal or informal nature of different cultures impact business communication?

Formal cultures tend to be organized in hierarchies according to status and power, while informal cultures value egalitarian attitudes with smaller differences in status and power. These contrasting values determine how someone should respond to people of higher status and can cause conflict in a business relationship.

People from formal cultures may be offended by the easy familiarity of their contacts from informal cultures; whereas, those from informal cultures may see their formal contacts as distant, stuffy, pompous, or arrogant. Misunderstandings can be avoided if both sides are aware that different business behaviors result from different cultural values rather than individual idiosyncrasies (Gesteland, 2005).

What are some examples of countries with formal cultures?

Examples of countries with hierarchical cultures would be most of Europe and Asia, the Mediterranean region, the Middle East, and Latin America.

TIP

When in an unfamiliar situation, it is better to err on the side of formality.

What are some examples of informal cultures?

Examples of egalitarian cultures include the United States, Canada, Australia, New Zealand, Nordic countries, and the Netherlands.

What are some ways to show respect to people from formal cultures?

Recognize that status differences are important in formal cultures, which you might demonstrate in the following ways:

✳ Address people in a formal manner (Ms., Mrs., Dr., Mr., etc.) using their last names until you are invited to use first names. Note that you may never be invited to use first names. Titles, such as Doctor and Professor are highly valued in many cultures (Pagana, 2009).

✳ Acknowledge and respect differences in status. For example, if doing business in Thailand, shake hands with your business associates, but not with their domestic workers.

✳ Make sure your clothes demonstrate respect and show proper deference. For example, men should wear a suit and tie when meeting—even during a hot season. If the air conditioner does not work, keeping suit jackets on shows respect.

"A traveler of taste will notice that the wise are polite all over the world, but the fool only at home."

–Oliver Goldsmith

Deal-Focused and Relationship-Focused Cultures

How important is relationship building for establishing business connections?

In the majority of the world's business relationships, a relationship-focused (RF) approach is the norm. This means that RF people prefer to deal with people they can trust, such as family, friends, and organizations known to them. They try to avoid doing business with strangers.

Comparatively, cultures open to doing business with strangers are deal-focused. The interested person can usually make an initial contact without having a previous relationship or connection. A referral is helpful, but not necessary. This difference is important to consider from the beginning and throughout any business relationship.

What are some examples of countries that are relationship focused?

Good examples include the Middle East, most of Africa, Latin America, and the Asia/Pacific region (Gesteland, 2005).

What are some examples of countries that are deal focused?

Strong deal-focused approaches are seen mainly in northern Europe, North America, Australia, and New Zealand (Gesteland, 2005). For example, most Americans are open to discussing business with people they don't know.

Do you have any suggestions to initiate a business connection in a relationship-based culture?

The best thing to do is to arrange to be introduced by an intermediary. A third-party introduction bridges the relationship gap between you and the other person. For example, in China, a business relationship can only be initiated if you know the right people; or you can arrange an introduction by using someone else's personal connections.

What are some tips for dealing with contacts from relationship-based cultures?

These people won't do business until they know and trust you; therefore, don't expect to accomplish your goals in one quick meeting. You need to make a friend before you make a deal. Here are some guidelines:

* Allow plenty of time: Forming a business relationship may require several meetings before getting down to specifics.

* Engage in small talk: A lot of time is needed to get to know one another and build a relationship.

* Be prepared to socialize with your new contacts: Important information is exchanged over a drink or a meal (Carte & Fox, 2004).

TIP

In many parts of the world, a five iron (golf club) closes a culture gap faster than a fifth of Scotch (Gesteland, 2005).

Communication Coach

It took Volkswagen more than 9 years to negotiate with the government of China to open an automobile factory in Shanghai (Gesteland, 2005).

Lesson: Building trust and developing a relationship takes a long time in relationship-focused cultures.

What are some tips for dealing with contacts from deal-focused cultures?

Be prepared to get down to business after only a few minutes of small talk. You can learn most of what you need to know in days rather than in weeks or months. Socialization can take place over drinks, meals, or sports. Rapport is also built when working out agreements.

After a business relationship is initiated, is there a difference in communication between the deal-focused and relationship-focused cultures?

Yes. Deal-oriented negotiators tend to value a direct, straightforward language, while relationship-focused negotiators favor an indirect, roundabout style. This can cause a lot of confusion because people from different cultures can expect different outcomes from the communication (Gesteland, 2005).

When communicating with others, a priority for deal-focused business people is to be clearly understood. They usually mean what they say and say what they mean. For example, German negotiators are known for their frank, and sometimes blunt, language. Directness and frankness is equated with sincerity and honesty.

Relationship-focused business people give priority to maintaining harmony and promoting smooth interpersonal relationships. They are careful about what they say and try to avoid embarrassing or offending others. For example, most Japanese, Chinese, or Southeast Asians don't like to use the word "No." To avoid insulting someone, they may say, "We will have to give that further study," "That would be difficult," "Maybe," or "That might be inconvenient." In relationship-focused cultures, directness and frankness are equated with immaturity and naiveté—even arrogance (Gesteland, 2005).

Is communication impacted by context?

Yes. In relationship-focused cultures, the meaning of the message is often found in the context surrounding the words rather than the words themselves. The polite communication of Asian, Middle Easterners, Africans, and Latinos tends to be implicit and highly contextual. They expect you to be able to interpret what they mean from what you know about cultural values, their tone, and their body language.

Low-context communicators tend to express themselves in concrete, explicit, and unequivocal terms. What they say is what they mean. Americans, Scandinavians, Finns, and Germans are low-context communicators.

Do you have any suggestions for communicating with highly contextual speakers?

Here are some tips for high-context communicators:

* Don't take what they say literally. For example, if a Japanese colleague says something is "difficult," he's probably saying it is impossible. Pay attention to his eyes and body language. Wait. Listen.

* Don't get irritated if you find it hard to grasp the message. Burying the message in circular talk comes naturally to high-context communicators. Be patient, listen hard, and read between the lines. Ask questions to verify correct understanding (Carte & Fox, 2004).

Do you have any suggestions for communicating with low-context speakers?

Here are some tips for low-context communicators:

* Take what they say literally. For example, if an American says something is "difficult," he means it is difficult, not impossible.

* Don't be offended if they openly disagree with you. They are not being insensitive or aggressive. They are trying to be clear and unequivocal to show respect and honesty (Gesteland, 2005).

Communication Coach

When Richard lived in Singapore, he and his wife hired a tutor to learn Mandarin. When his parents both died within a few weeks, he missed a month of lessons while attending funerals in Wisconsin. When he returned, his tutor asked why he had missed a month's worth of lessons. Suffering from grief and exhaustion, he blurted out that both of his parents had just died. After a look of surprise, the tutor suddenly laughed out loud and giggled for several seconds. Although, intellectually, this response was not unexpected, Richard felt as though he had been punched in the stomach.

Lesson: People from certain Asian cultures hide their nervousness, embarrassment, or stress behind laughter.

Gestures and Nonverbal Communication

How should you handle gestures in communicating with people from other cultures?

Very carefully. Several gestures can be misunderstood or considered insulting. Here are some ambiguous gestures to avoid (Gesteland, 2005; Martin & Chaney, 2006; Pagana, 2008; Pagana, 2009):

* The "okay" sign (making a circle with the thumb and forefinger and having three raised fingers) is offensive in many countries, such as Brazil. Additionally, the gesture means "money" in Japan and "worthless" in France.

* "Thumbs up" sign: Although it means "great" in many parts of the world, it is a rude sexual sign in Egypt.

* "V" for victory sign, especially with the palm facing inward: This is offensive in Great Britain.

* Pointing with the index finger is rude throughout East and Southeast Asia.

* Waving your hand with your arm raised may be misunderstood as "no."

* Beckoning with the index finger is reserved for calling dogs and prostitutes in many parts of Asia.

* Fist in palm: This is considered an obscene sexual gesture in Southeast Asia.

* Left hand: The left hand is considered unclean in Muslim, Hindu, and Buddhist cultures. Avoid touching people or objects with the left hand.

* Tapping your head: The means different things to many Europeans. For example, tapping your forehead in France, Italy, and Germany while looking at someone implies, "Hey, you are stupid." The same gesture in Spain and Great Britain means, "I am so clever!"

* Showing the sole of your shoe: The bottom of the shoe or the foot is considered unclean in some cultures. Avoid crossing your legs and making the sole visible to others.

* Placing your hands on your hips: This gesture suggests aggressiveness and can imply you are making a challenge in such countries as Mexico and Argentina.

* Standing with your arms folded: This is viewed as arrogant in France.

* Putting your hand on your stomach: In Italy, this gesture shows your dislike of someone.

* Winking at a person: This is inappropriate in many countries, such as Australia and Taiwan.

In many parts of the world, people raise their eyebrows during communication. What is the significance of this expression?

This expression can also have different meanings in different cultures. Table 10.1 shows examples (Gesteland, 2005, p.81):

10.1 Interpretation of Raised Eyebrows in Different Parts of the World	
CULTURE	*INTERPRETATION*
United States	Interest, surprise
China	Disagreement
Middle Eastern	"No!"
Germany	"You are clever."
The Philippines	"Hello!"

Does nodding the head usually imply agreement?

No. In the United States, we think that when people nod, they are agreeing with us. However, in Southeast Asia, nodding means, "I hear you," not "I agree with you." Direct agreement is not a cultural norm, so members of these cultural groups may nod instead of voicing disagreement. Nodding by a Vietnamese person may indicate respect for the speaker rather than agreement and understanding. American Eskimos seldom disagree with others in public. Even if they disagree, they nod "yes" just to be polite (Giger & Davidhizar, 2008).

How does eye contact impact communication?

Eye contact must be interpreted within its cultural context to optimize communication. People are usually confused when others use more or less eye contact than they do.

In the United States, it is polite to look someone in the eye. This demonstrates openness, sincerity, trustworthiness, and confidence (Pagana, 2008). However, in many Asian countries, a person of lower status may avoid eye contact with persons of higher status or educational backgrounds (Purnell & Paulanka, 2008). Looking away is a sign of respect. Here are samples of implications in different countries:

* Mexico: Continued, intense eye contact is considered aggressive and threatening.

* Japan: Prolonged eye contact is not the norm. Looking people directly in the eye invades their privacy.

* France: Don't be surprised if you may be looked at more intensely than expected.

* Great Britain: Often, the British do not look the person directly in the eye or maintain eye contact when talking. Don't be offended (Morrison & Conaway, 2006).

Is smiling a universal gesture of happiness?

Not necessarily. Most Americans smile easily as a gesture of happiness. However, in the Japanese culture, if you feel truly happy, you do not need to smile (Purnell & Paulanka, 2008). Note that people can also use facial expressions to convey an emotion opposite to what they are feeling. For example, in Asia, people may conceal negative emotions with a smile. People from Japan and China may smile when they are embarrassed or confused (Giger & Davidhizar, 2008).

"No act of kindness, no matter how small, is ever wasted."

–Aesop

Personal Space

How do you handle personal-space issues when interacting with international colleagues?

Treat the area near a person's body with care. Some people describe personal space as the expandable bubble people carry with them. This bubble can expand or contract based on the closeness of others in the environment (Richmond & McCroskey, 2009). Be aware that proximity when conversing with someone is dictated by culture. We can unknowingly offend others by moving closer or farther away when speaking. Violating someone's personal space can lead to interpersonal stress and anger (Leininger & McFarland, 2002).

The concept of group rights has an impact on space. Cultures that give priority to the individual (the United States, Canada, and Northern and Western Europe) rather than the group are more likely to value privacy. People from these cultures may feel uncomfortable when forced to sit or stand close to people they do not know well.

In cultures that give priority to the group (Asian, Latino, Mediterranean, and most Middle Eastern cultures) rather than the individual, group rights and shared space are important considerations. People from these cultures welcome physical closeness and may prefer to stand close to one another when holding a conversation. In some of these cultures, men kissing or holding hands with each other is normal. Rejecting these signs can make you seem discourteous and cold (Giger & Davidhizar, 2008: Munoz & Luckmann, 2005).

Can you give some examples of how far apart people in different cultures stand when talking?

People in the United States usually stand about 3 feet apart when speaking. The distance of comfort is more than 3 feet in Japan. The British maintain a wide personal space between conversation partners. In Italy, Mexico, and Argentina, the distance is closer. Chilean people stand closer than many Northern Europeans, North Americans, or Asians. When talking with Chileans, try not to back away. If you do, they will probably step closer and close the gap (Morrison & Conaway, 2006).

Communication Coach

I will never forget the time I visited my daughter when she was spending a semester abroad in India. One day we traveled by local bus to visit an orphanage where she worked. We were packed into the bus with people touching us on all sides. The children in front of me were inches from my face and commenting on my "cat eyes" (blue eyes). Recognizing my extreme discomfort, my daughter instructed me to put my backpack up in front of my face.

Lesson: Because I am from the United States, my sense of privacy was violated on the crowded bus. Physical closeness is not a problem with Indian people.

Gift Giving

If you are attending a dinner at someone's house, should you bring a gift?

Gift giving is an important custom. If dining at someone's house, you should bring a gift for the hostess. However, what you consider a nice gift may not be the right gift. For example, expensive gifts in China may be considered a bribe. Exchange gifts with the right hand in the Middle East because the left hand is used for hygiene and is considered unclean (Leininger & McFarland,2002; Pagana, 2008).

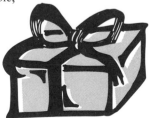

How can you give the right gift?

This requires research. Some gifts can have a negative meaning. For example, a clock is associated with funerals in China, red flowers are for lovers in Germany, and yellow flowers symbolize death in Mexico. Don't give gifts made of silver in Mexico because of a negative association with the trinkets sold to tourists (Morrison & Conaway, 2006). Examples of gifts that are usually acceptable include nice pens, chocolates, toys for children, local crafts from your area, or illustrated books from your country.

Gift giving is a refined art with many symbolic meanings in Japan. Seek guidance from an advisor or Japanese friend. For example, gifts should be wrapped with lightly tinted paper, not white paper, which symbolizes death. Gifts are given and received with both hands and are opened after the donor has departed.

What if the person refuses to accept your gift?

In some cultures, such as Korea, the gift will not be accepted initially. The refusal is part of the ritual. Be persistent until it is accepted.

Should you open a gift when you receive it?

In some countries, the gift is opened when it is received, and in others, it is opened later. For example, in China, the gift is not opened when it is received to demonstrate that the giving of the gift is more valuable than the actual item (Pachter, 2006).

Shaking Hands

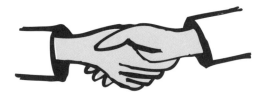

How does handshake etiquette differ across cultures?

The handshake is the most common form of physical contact among business people around the world; therefore, very important in the communication process. How you shake hands sends different signals to different people. For example, in the United States, a firm handshake is used to communicate confidence and self-assurance. Don't judge other cultures by their handshakes. Here are some points to consider:

* Who should initiate the handshake? (It may be the most senior person.)

* Should men wait for women to extent their hand? (In many European countries, yes.)

* Can a man shake a woman's hand? (Not if he is Muslim or Hindu.)

* Should the grip be gentle or firm? (See Table 10.2.)

 Handshake Variations Throughout the World

North America	Firm and infrequent
Latin America	Firm and frequent
Great Britain	Moderate firmness
Germany	Firm, brisk, and frequent
France	Light, quick, and frequent
Denmark	Firm and brief
Ireland	Firm and brief
Middle East	Gentle, repeated, and lingering
South Asia	Gentle, often lingering
Korea	Moderately firm
Most of Asia	Very gentle and infrequent

(Gesteland, 2005; Pagana, 2008)

Are there gender differences in handshake etiquette?

Different customs are seen throughout the world. For example, in India and Saudi Arabia, the handshake is only between men. In Germany, men should wait for the woman to extend her hand for the handshake.

Is the bow the equivalent of a handshake?

Yes, in Japan and China, the bow is used instead of the handshake as a greeting.

If a bow is used instead of a handshake, who bows first?

In a rank-conscious society, such as Japan, the person of lower rank bows first and lowest.

What should you do if someone ignores your handshake?

Gently drop your hand to your side. Many cultural preferences and sensitivities affect the handshake. For example, in the Hindu culture, contact between men and women is avoided; therefore, men do not shake hands with women. There also may be physical limitations or sickness issues.

How do you know how to greet an international business associate?

If you are not sure how to greet the person, start with a handshake or follow his or her lead. If the person greets you with a kiss, follow suit. You may offend the person if you pull away. A bow or hug may be appropriate in some cultures.

✔ *Checklist*

Cross-cultural Communication

❑ Did I consider my colleague's time orientation?

❑ Do I know if my colleague is from an emotionally expressive or reserved culture?

❑ Do I know how to deal with conversational silence?

❑ Have I considered differences in status?

❑ Am I prepared to err on the side of formality?

❑ Do I need a referral to make an initial connection with a potential contact?

❑ Did I determine whether my colleague is from a deal-focused or relationship-focused culture?

❑ Do I know if my colleague favors direct, straightforward language or an indirect, roundabout style?

❑ Am I aware of gestures that may have ambiguous meanings?

❑ If my colleague nods her head, do I know the meaning of this expression?

❑ Am I prepared to handle personal space issues without offending anyone?

Frequently Asked Questions

 If you have a meeting scheduled for 10 a.m. in a polychronic culture, what time should you arrive?

Even though the meeting will probably start late, show your respect by being on time. Bring something to read while you wait. The visitor is expected to acquiesce to local customs.

 If doing business in a Muslim country, how does a left-handed person handle signing a document?

The person can sign the document with the left hand, but should hand the document to others using the right hand.

 How can you use information about cultural generalizations to avoid stereotyping?

A generalization is a statement about trends or patterns within a group, which can serve as a starting point for understanding others. You should gather further information to determine whether the generalization applies to a particular person. People are unique and should not be stereotyped. Differences exist in every culture. A cultural stereotype assumes that all people of a certain group are alike. A stereotype is an ending point with no effort to consider individual differences.

 If you do not understand why someone from a different culture does or says something, is it acceptable to ask him or her?

Yes, polite questions demonstrate an interest in another culture and help build relationships.

Should humor be used when communicating with people from other cultures?

When people are from a different culture, the use of humor should be limited and deliberate because humor can be an obstacle to a relationship if misunderstood.

 Are there any guidelines for working with translators?

Yes. Look at and speak directly to the person instead of to the translator. Be careful of telling jokes, because humor does not translate well.

 If you are communicating with international colleagues and you think you have offended someone, what should you do?

Your mistake may be obvious from someone's comments, expression, or body language. Apologize immediately. If you don't know what caused the offense, say, "Please help me. Tell me what I did, so I won't do it again." Demonstrate a humble and respectful attitude.

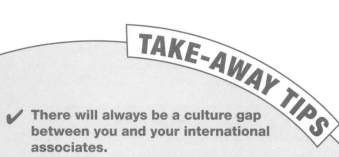

TAKE-AWAY TIPS

✔ **There will always be a culture gap between you and your international associates.**

✔ **Find out as much as you can about cultural values and what lies behind beliefs.**

✔ **Behavior which is polite and proper in one culture may be offensive and rude in another.**

✔ **When conducting international business, choose the cultural approach that best fits the local circumstances.**

✔ **Remind yourself that the way you do things in your part of the world is not universal.**

✔ **Punctuality can vary according to whether the engagement is business or social. For example, a business meeting in a polychronic culture may start 10 minutes late—and a wedding reception may begin 2 hours late!**

✔ **Your communication efforts can fail if you are nonverbally illiterate—unaware of the importance of gestures and other body language.**

✔ **Look at situations across cultures as "different" rather than right or wrong.**

References

Front matter

Adubato, S. (2007). *Make the connection: Improve your communication skills at home and at work.* Barnes & Noble Publisher.

Blalock, M. (2005). Listen up: Why good communication is good business. Retrieved July 29, 2009 from http://www.bus.wisc.edu/update/winter05/business_communication.asp

Chapter 1

Acuff, J. & Woods, W. (2004). *The relationship edge in business: Connecting with customers and colleagues when it counts.* Hoboken, NJ: John Wiley & Sons.

Dykes, P., Cashen, M., Foster, M., Gallagher, J., Kennedy, M., MacCallum, R. et al (2006). Surveying acute care providers in the U.S. to explore the impact of HIT on the role of nurses and interdisciplinary communication in acute health care settings. *Journal of Healthcare Information Management, 20*(2), pp. 36-44.

Eichhorn, K. C., Thomas-Maddox, C., & Wanzer, M. B. (2008). *Interpersonal communication: Building rewarding relationships.* Dubuque, Iowa: Kendall/Hunt Publishing Company.

Evans, G. (2003). *She wins, you win: The most important rule every businesswoman needs to know.* New York: Gotham Books.

Heinemann, G. D. & Zeiss, A. M. (eds.) (2002). *Team performance in health care: Assessment and development.* New York: Plenum.

Kintish, W. (2006). *I hate networking: Discover the secrets of confident and effective networkers.* Manchester, Ontario: JAM Publications.

Kirchheimer, B. (2010). Study: RN-doctor communication better. Retrieved July 27, 2010 from http://news.nurse.com/apps/pbcs.dll/article?AID=/20100111/NE02/301110005&template=printarttMagnetHospitals.

Klaus, P. (2007). *The hard truth about soft skills: Workplace lessons smart people wish they'd learned sooner.* New York: Collins.

Kramer, M. & Schmalenberg, C. (2008). Confirmation of a healthy work environment. *Critical Care Nurse, 28* (2), 56-63.

Lindeke, L. L. & Sieckert, A. M. (2005). Nurse-physician workplace collaboration. *Online Journal of Issues in Nursing, 10*(1). Retrieved June 17, 2010 from http://www.nursingworld.org/MainMenuCategories/ANA-Marketplace/ANAPeriodicals/OJIN/TableofContents/Volume102005/No1Jan05/tpc26_416011.aspx

Lindsell-Roberts, S. (2000). *Business professionals kit for dummies.* New York: IDG Books.

Maxwell, J. C. (2007). *Talent is never enough: Discover the choices that will take you beyond your talent.* Nashville, TN: Thomas Nelson.

Pagana, K. (2008). *The nurse's etiquette advantage: How professional etiquette can advance your nursing career.* Indianapolis, IN: Sigma Theta Tau International Honor Society of Nursing.

Rafferty, A.M., Ball, J., & Aiken, H. (2001). Are teamwork and professional autonomy compatible, and do they result in improved health care? *Quality in Health Care, 10* (Suppl II), ii32-ii37.

Reader, T.W., Flin R., Mearns, K. & Cuthbertson, B.H. (2007). Interdisciplinary communication in the intensive care unit. *British Journal of Anaesthesia, 98* (3), 347-352.

RoAnn, S. (2000). *How to work a room: The ultimate guide to savvy socializing in person and online.* New York: Quill.

Shepard, M.D. & Stimmler, J.K. (2005). *Stop the whining & start winning.* New York: Penguin Group.

Shipley, D. & Schwalbe, W. (2007). *Send: The essential guide to email for office and home.* New York: Alfred A. Knopf.

Soden, F. (1996). *Hook spin buzz: How to command attention, change minds, and influence people.* Princeton: Peterson's/Pacesetter Books.

Tannen, D. (1994). *Talking from 9 to 5: How women's and men's conversational styles affect who gets heard, who gets credit, and what gets done at work.* New York: William Morrow and Company, Inc.

Tannen, D. (1990). *You just don't understand: Women and men in conversation.* New York: William Morrow.

Chapter 2

Brody, M. (2008). *Speaking is an audience-centered sport* (4th ed.). Jenkintown, PA: Career Skills Press.

Denning, S. (2001). *The springboard: How storytelling ignites action in knowledge-era organizations.* Woburn, MA: KMCI Press.

Lindsell-Roberts, S. (2000). *Business professionals kit for dummies.* New York: IDG Books.

Steele, W. R. (2009). *Presentation skills 201: How to take it to the next level as a confident and engaging presenter.* Denver: Outskirts Press, Inc.

Stevenson, D. (2009). *Personal communication. Doug Stevenson's Story Theatre Method.* Retrieved June 17, 2010 from www.storytelling-in-business.com

Weissman, J. (2005). *Absolute beginner's guide to winning presentations.* Indianapolis, IN: QUE Publishing.

Chapter 3

Brody, M. (2008). *Speaking is an audience-centered sport* (4th ed.). Jenkintown, PA: Career Skills Press.

Carnegie, D. (n.d.) Retrieved June 18, 2010 from www.communispond.com/resources/uploads/echo/02-28-07.pdf

Chaney, L. H., & Martin, J. S. (2007). *The essential guide to business etiquette.* Westport, CT: Praeger Publishers.

Detz, J. (2000). *It's not what you say, it's how you say it.* New York: St. Martin's Press.

Gottesman, D., & Mauro, B. (2001). *Taking center stage: Masterful public speaking using acting skills you never knew you had.* New York: Berkley Books.

Steele, W. R. (2009). *Presentation skills 201: How to take it to the next level as a confident and engaging presenter.* Denver, CO: Outskirts Press, Inc.

Weissman, J. (2005). *Absolute beginner's guide to winning presentations.* Indianapolis, IN: QUE Publishing.

Yate, M., & Sander, P. (2003). *Knock 'em dead business presentations.* Avon, MA: Adams Media Corporation.

Chapter 4

Chaney, L. H., & Martin, J. S. (2007). *The essential guide to business etiquette.* Westport, CT: Praeger Publishers.

Lindsell-Roberts, S. (2004). *Strategic business letters and e-mail.* New York: Houghton Mifflin Company.

Lindsell-Roberts, S. (2000). *Business Professionals Kit For Dummies.* New York: IDG Books.

Pagana, K. (2008). *The nurse's etiquette advantage: How professional etiquette can advance your nursing career.* Indianapolis, IN: Sigma Theta Tau International.

Post, P. (Peggy), & Post, P. (Peter) (1999). *The etiquette advantage in business: Personal skills for professional success.* New York: HarperCollins Books.

Chapter 5

Chaney, L. H., & Martin, J. S. (2007). *The essential guide to business etiquette.* Westport, CT: Praeger Publishers.

Eichhorn, K. C., Thomas-Maddox, C., & Wanzer, M. B. (2008). *Interpersonal communication: Building rewarding relationships*. Dubuque, Iowa: Kendall/Hunt Publishing Company.

Lindsell-Roberts, S. (2000). *Business professionals kit for dummies*. New York: IDG Books.

Lindsell-Roberts, S. (2004). *Strategic business letters and e-mail*. New York: Houghton Mifflin Company.

Pagana, K. (2008). *The nurse's etiquette advantage: How professional etiquette can advance your nursing career*. Indianapolis, IN: Sigma Theta Tau International.

Post, P. (Peggy), & Post, P. (Peter) (1999). *The etiquette advantage in business: Personal skills for professional success*. New York: HarperCollins Books.

Robbins, S. P. (2003). *Essentials of organizational behavior* (7th ed.). Upper Saddle River, New Jersey: Prentice Hall.

Shipley, D., & Schwalbe, W. (2007). *Send: The essential guide to e-mail for office and home*. New York: Alfred A. Knopf.

Chapter 6

Duff, D. (2001). Writing for publication. *AXON, 22* (4), 36-39.

Johnstone, M. (2004). *Effective writing for health professionals: A practical guide to getting published*. New York: Routledge.

Northam, S., Trubenbach, M., & Bentov, L. (2000). Nursing journal survey: Information to help you publish. *Nurse Educator, 25*(5), 227-236.

Northam, S., Yarbrough, S., Haas, B., & Duke, G. (2010). Journal editor survey: Information to help authors publish. *Nurse Editor, 35*(1), 29-36.

Oermann, M. (2002). *Writing for publication in nursing*. Philadelphia: Lippincott.

Pagana, K. (1989). Writing strategies to demystify publishing. *Journal of Continuing Education in Nursing, 20*(2), 58-63.

Pierce, L. (2009). Writing for publication: You can do it! *Rehabilitation Nursing, 34*(1), 3-8.

Plaisance, L. (2003). The "write" way to get published in a professional journal. *Pain Management Nursing, 4*(4), 165-170.

Ruth-Sahd, L., & King, C. (2006). A diamond in the rough, to a polished gemstone ring: Writing for publication in a nursing journal. *Dimensions Critical Care Nursing, 25*(3), 113-120.

Schilling, L. (2005). Publish or perish: Writing under pressure. *Pediatric Nursing, 31*(3), 234, 236.

Wills, C. (2000). Strategies for managing barriers to the writing process. *Nursing Forum, 35*(4), 5-13.

Wink, D. (2002). Writing to get published. *Nephrology Nursing Journal, 29*(5), 461-467.

Chapter 7

Adubato, S. (2006). *Make the connection: Improve your communication at work and at home.* New Brunswick, NJ: Rivergate Books.

Beebe, S. A., & Masterson, JT (2000). *Communicating in small groups: Principles and practices* (6th ed.). New York: Longman Publishing.

Booher, D. (1994). *Communicate with confidence: How to say it right the first time and every time.* New York: McGraw-Hill, Inc.

Brody, M. (2005). *Professional impressions: Etiquette for everyone, every day* (3rd ed.). Jenkintown, PA: Career Skills Press.

Chaney, L. H., & Martin, J. S. (2007). *The essential guide to business etiquette.* Westport, CT: Praeger Publishers.

Lindsell-Roberts, S. (2000). *Business professionals kit for dummies.* New York: IDG Books.

Pagana, K. (2008). *The nurse's etiquette advantage: How professional etiquette can advance your nursing career.* Indianapolis, IN: Sigma Theta Tau International.

Post, P. (Peggy) & Post, P. (Peter) (1999). *The etiquette advantage in business: Personal skills for professional success.* New York: HarperCollins Publications

Schindler, E. (2008). Running an effective teleconference or virtual meeting. Retrieved October 10, 2009, from http://cio.com/article/print/184550

Chapter 8

Alsop, R. *The trophy kids grow up: How the millennial generation is shaking up the workplace.* San Francisco: Jossey-Bass.

Anonymous. (2009). Few workers use social media tools at their job. (2009). *Information Outlook*, 13(8), 7. Retrieved February 1, 2010 from http://www.thefreelibrary.com/Few+workers+use+social+media+tools+at+their+job.-a0215324835.

Bolte Taylor, J. (2007). *My Stroke of Insight: A brain scientist's personal journey.* New York: Viking Press.

HCPro, Inc. (2009). Bridging the generation gap with diverse, creative education. *Strategies for Nurse Managers*, 9(11), 1-3. Retrieved February 2, 2010 from http://www.strategiesfornursemanagers.com/ce_detail/245426.cfm.

Coates, J. (2006). *Generational learning styles.* River Falls, WI: LERN Books.

Erickson, T. (2008). *Plugged in: The Generation Y guide to thriving at work.* Boston, MA: Harvard Business Press.

Galinsky, E., Aumann, K., & Bond, J. T. 2009. *Times are changing: Gender and generation at work and at home*. New York: Families and Work Institute. Retrieved February 1, 2010 from http://familiesandwork.org/site/research/reports/Times_Are_Changing.pdf

Glennon, T. J. (2009). Millennials in the workforce: Implications for managers. *Administration & Management Special Interest Section Quarterly / American Occupational Therapy Association, 25*(1), 1-4.

Hobbs, J. L., Hostvedt, K., White, P., Benavente, V., Brooks, M., Poghosyan, L., et al. (2005, November). *Generations: A walk through the past, present and future*. Paper presented at the meeting of the Sigma Theta Tau Biennial Convention. Indianapolis, Indiana.

Hannon, B. (2009, July). Addressing intergenerational conflict in the workplace. *HCPro's Advisor to the ANCC Magnet Recognition Program, 5*(7), 6.

Howe, N., & Strauss, W. (1992). *Generations: The history of America's future, 1584 to 2069*. New York: Harper Perennial.

Kramer, L.W. (2010). Generational diversity. *Critical Care Nursing, 29*(3):125-128.

Lower, J. (2007). Brace yourself for Generation Y nurses. *American Nurse Today, 2*(8):26-29.

Pardue, K. T., & Morgan, P. (2008). Millennials considered: A new generation, new approaches, and implications for nursing education. *Nursing Education Perspectives, 29*(2), 74-79.

Pew Internet & American Life Project. (2009). Pew internet Project Data Memo from January 14, 2009.

Prensky, M. (2001). Digital natives, digital immigrants. *On the Horizon, 9*(5), 1-6.

Rainie, L. (2009). Teens in the digital age. Retrieved February 1, 2010 from http://www.slideshare.net/PewInternet/teens-in-digital-age

RainmakerThinking. (2007). Executive summary: Managing the generation mix 2007: An update on the research of RainmakerThinking conducted since 1993. Retrieved February 2, 2010 from http://www.rainmakerthinking.com/reports_and_white_papers.php.

Rollins, G. (2008). CNO Burnout. *Hospitals & Health Networks*. Retrieved February 1, 2010 from http://www.hhnmag.com/hhnmag_app/jsp/articledisplay.jsp?dcrpath=HHNMAG/Article/data/04APR2008/0804HHN_FEA_CoverStory&domain=HHNMAG

Saver, C. (2010). Tweeting, posting, and yammering: Social media in the OR. *OR Manager, 26*(2):1,12-14.

Sherman, R.O. (2006). Leading a multigenerational nursing workforce: Issues, challenges and strategies. *Online Journal of Issues in Nursing, 11*(2). Retrieved February 1, 2010 from http://www.nursingworld.org/MainMenuCategories/ANAMarketplace/ANAPeriodicals/OJIN/TableofContents/Volume112006/No2May06/tpc30_216074.aspx.

Siela, D. (2006). Managing the multigenerational nursing staff. *American Nurse Today, 1*(3):47-49.

Stanton Smith, W. (2008). *Decoding generational differences: Fact, fiction ... or should we just get back to work?* New York. Deloitte Development LLC.

Sudheimer, E. (2009). Appreciating both sides of the generation gap: Baby Boomer and generation X nurses working together. *Nursing Forum, 44*(1), 57-63.

Twenge, J. M. (2006). *Generation me: Why today's young Americans are more confident, assertive, entitled—and more miserable than ever before.* New York: Free Press.

Weston, M. J. (2006). Integrating generational perspectives in nursing. *Online Journal of Issues in Nursing, 11*(2). Retrieved February 1, 2010 from http://www.nursingworld.org/MainMenuCategories/ANAMarketplace/ANAPeriodicals/OJIN/TableofContents/Volume112006/No2May06/tpc30_116073.aspx.

Wieck, K., Dols, J., & Northam, S. (2009). What nurses want: The nurse incentives project. *Nursing Economics, 27*(3), 169-177, 201.

Wilson, B., Squires, M., Widger, K., Cranley, L., & Tourangeau, A. (2008). Job satisfaction among a multigenerational workforce. *Journal of Nursing Management, 16,* 716-723.

Winograd, M., & Hais, M. D. (2008). *Millennial makeover: MySpace, YouTube & the future of American politics.* Piscataway, NJ: Rutgers University Press.

Chapter 9

Berkman, R. (2008). *The art of strategic listening: Finding market intelligence through blogs and other social media.* Ithaca, NY: Paramount Market Publishing, Inc.

Boyd, D. M., & Ellison, N. B. (2007). Social network sites: Definition, history, and scholarship. *Journal of Computer-Mediated Communication, 13*(1), article 11. Retrieved March 1, 2010 from http//jcmc.indiana.edu/vol13/issue1/boyd.ellison.html

Holtz, S., & Demopoulos, T. (2006). *Blogging for business: Everything you need to know and why you should care.* Chicago: Kaplan Publishing.

Liburdi, M. C. (2008). Working it! : How to make the most out of social networking to enhance career prospects. *NSNA Imprint, 55*(4), 62-70.

Magg, M. (2005). The potential use of "blogs" in nursing education. *Computers, Informatics, Nursing, 23*(1), 16-24.

Safko, L., & Brake, D. (2009). *The social media bible: Tactics, tools, & strategies for business success.* Hoboken, New Jersey: John Wiley & Sons.

Saver, C. (2010). Tweeting, posting, and yammering: Social media in the OR. *OR Manager, 26*(2):1, 12-4.

Scott, D. M. (2009). *The new rules of marketing and PR.* Hoboken, NJ: John Wiley & Sons.

Weil, D. (2006). *The corporate blogging book: Absolutely everything you need to know to get it right.* New York: Penguin Group.

Chapter 10

Carte, P., & Fox, C. (2004). *Bridging the culture gap: A practical guide to international business communication.* Sterling, VA: Kogan Page.

Gesteland, R. (2005). *Cross-cultural business behavior: Negotiating, selling, sourcing, and managing across cultures* (4th ed.). Hendon, VA: Copenhagen Business School Press.

Giger, J. N., Davidhizar, R. E. (2008). *Transcultural nursing: Assessment and intervention* (5th ed.). St Louis: Mosby/ Elsevier.

Leininger, M., & McFarland, M. R. (2002). *Transcultural nursing: Concepts, theories, research, and practice* (3rd ed.). New York: McGraw-Hill.

Martin, J., & Chaney, L. (2006). *Global business etiquette: A guide to international communication and customs.* Westwood, CT: Praeger.

Morrison, R., & Conaway, W. A. (2006). *Kiss, bow, or shake hands: The best-selling guide to doing business in more than 60 countries* (2nd ed.) Avon, MA: Adams Media.

Munoz, C., & Luckmann, J. (2005). *Transcultural communication in nursing* (2nd ed.) Clifton Park, NY: Thomson Delmar.

Pachter, B. (2006). *When the little things count: And they always count.* New York: Marlowe & Company.

Pagana, K. D. (2009). Mind your manners...multiculturally. *Nurse Week, 10*(7), 18-23.

Pagana, K. (2008). *The nurse's etiquette advantage: How professional etiquette can advance your nursing career.* Indianapolis, IN: Sigma Theta Tau International.

Purnell, L. D., & Paulanka, B. J. (2008). *Transcultural health care: A culturally competent approach,* (3rd ed.). Philadelphia: F.A. Davis Company.

Richmond, V. P., & McCroskey, J. C. (2009). *Organizational communication for survival: Making work, work* (4th ed.) Boston: Pearson Education, Inc.

Index

N–O

P

Business Communication Quiz Answers

✳

1. True. Participation in sports provides many lessons about the importance of teamwork.

2. True. Women usually want empathy, while men want advice to fix the problem.

3. False. That is boring. Start with something to grab the audience's attention.

4. False. The story is an asset only if it relates to the topic or illustrates a key point.

5. True. Use the "B" key.

6. True. People listed in the Bcc get the message but do not see the names and e-mail addresses of the other recipients. This protects their privacy.

7. False. Save them for informal correspondence with friends.

8. False. Review the author guidelines because some editors prefer a query letter and others do not.

9. False. There are specific criteria that must be met for listing someone as a co-author.

10. True. Don't waste people's time. Only hold a meeting if it is the best way to accomplish your goals.

11. True. They grew up with a lot of attention paid to them.

12. True. As an example, employers can learn where a candidate worked *previously* and for *whom* they worked.

13. True. Blogs are also more interactive.

14. False. Blogs get higher rankings on search engines than static websites.

15. True. When answered strategically, Twitter is a great example of social networking.

16. True. What you post on Facebook can have a negative impact on your career.

17. True. People view time and scheduling differently around the world.

18. False. It is an offensive gesture in many countries.

19. False. Not necessarily. In some cultures, people conceal negative emotions with a smile.

20. False. Some gifts have a negative meaning. The right gift requires a little research.